Thymectomy for Myasthenia Gravis

Editor

JOSHUA R. SONETT

THORACIC SURGERY CLINICS

www.thoracic.theclinics.com

Consulting Editor
M. BLAIR MARSHALL

May 2019 • Volume 29 • Number 2

ELSEVIER

1600 John F. Kennedy Boulevard • Suite 1800 • Philadelphia, Pennsylvania, 19103-2899

http://www.thoracic.theclinics.com

THORACIC SURGERY CLINICS Volume 29, Number 2
May 2019 ISSN 1547-4127, ISBN-13: 978-0-323-67829-2

Editor: John Vassallo (j.vassallo@elsevier.com)
Developmental Editor: Laura Fisher

Thoracic Surgery Clinics (ISSN 1547-4127) is published quarterly by Elsevier Inc., 360 Park Avenue South, New York, NY 10010-1710. Months of publication are February, May, August, and November. Business and editorial offices: 1600 John F. Kennedy Boulevard, Suite 1800, Philadelphia, PA 19103-2899. Periodicals postage paid at New York, NY, and additional mailing offices. Subscription prices are $382.00 per year (US individuals), $585.00 per year (US institutions), $100.00 per year (US students), $460.00 per year (Canadian individuals), $757.00 per year (Canadian institutions), $225.00 per year (Canadian and international students), $475.00 per year (international individuals), and $757.00 per year (international institutions). Foreign air speed delivery is included in all Clinics' subscription prices. All prices are subject to change without notice. **POSTMASTER:** Send address changes to Thoracic Surgery Clinics, Elsevier Health Sciences Division, Subscription Customer Service, 3251 Riverport Lane, Maryland Heights, MO 63043. **Customer Service (orders, claims, online, change of address): Telephone: 1-800-654-2452 (U.S. and Canada); 314-447-8871 (outside U.S. and Canada). Fax: 314-447-8029. E-mail: journalscustomerservice-usa@elsevier.com (for print support); journalsonlinesupport-usa@elsevier.com (for online support).**

Reprints. For copies of 100 or more, of articles in this publication, please contact Commercial Rights Department, Elsevier Inc., 360 Park Avenue South, New York, NY 10010-1710. Tel: 212-633-3874; Fax: 212-633-3820; E-mail: reprints@elsevier.com.

Thoracic Surgery Clinics is covered in *MEDLINE/PubMed (Index Medicus), EMBASE/Excerpta Medica, Science Citation Index Expanded (SciSearch®), Journal Citation Reports/Science Edition,* and *Current Contents®/Clinical Medicine.*

Contributors

CONSULTING EDITOR

M. BLAIR MARSHALL, MD, FACS
Chief, Division of Thoracic Surgery, Associate
Professor, Department of Surgery,
Georgetown University Medical Center,
Georgetown University School of Medicine,
Washington, DC, USA

EDITOR

JOSHUA R. SONETT, MD
Professor and Chief, Thoracic Surgery, Director,
Price Family Center for Comprehensive Chest
Care, Columbia University Irving Medical
Center, NewYork-Presbyterian Hospital, New
York, New York, USA

AUTHORS

VINCENZO AMBROGI, MD, PhD
Department of Surgical Sciences, Myasthenia
Gravis Multidisciplinary Program, Tor Vergata
University, Division of Thoracic Surgery, Tor
Vergata University Policlinic, Rome, Italy

BEATRICE ARAMINI, MD, PhD
Assistant Professor, Division of Thoracic
Surgery, Department of Medical and Surgical
Sciences for Children and Adults, University of
Modena and Reggio Emilia, Modena, Italy

GERO BAUER, MD
Department of Surgery, Competence Center of
Thoracic Surgery, Charité University Hospital
Berlin, Berlin, Germany

GIOVANNI M. COMACCHIO, MD
Thoracic Surgery Unit, Department of
Cardiologic, Thoracic and Vascular Sciences,
University Hospital, Padova, Italy

JOEL D. COOPER, MD
Professor of Surgery, Division of Thoracic
Surgery, University of Pennsylvania,
Philadelphia, Pennsylvania, USA

ARON ELSNER, MD
Department of Surgery, Competence Center of
Thoracic Surgery, Charité University Hospital
Berlin, Berlin, Germany

JIANG FAN, MD, PhD
Associate Professor, Department of Thoracic
Surgery, Shanghai Pulmonary Hospital, Tongji
University School of Medicine, Shanghai,
China

DONNA L. FARBER, PhD
Professor of Surgical Sciences, Department of
Surgery, Columbia Center for Translational
Immunology, Columbia University Irving
Medical Center, New York, New York, USA

MAHMOUD ISMAIL, MD
Department of Surgery, Competence Center of
Thoracic Surgery, Charité University Hospital
Berlin, Berlin, Germany

HENRY J. KAMINSKI, MD
Neumann Professor and Chair of Neurology,
Department of Neurology, George Washington
University, Washington, DC, USA

SHAF KESHAVJEE, MD
James Wallace McCutcheon Chair in
Surgery, Professor, Division of Thoracic
Surgery, Vice Chair, Innovation, Department
of Surgery, University of Toronto, Surgeon
in Chief, University Health Network, Toronto
General Hospital, Toronto, Ontario,
Canada

PHILIPPE H. LEMAÎTRE, MD
Clinical Fellow, Division of Thoracic Surgery,
Toronto General Hospital, University of
Toronto, Toronto, Ontario, Canada

FENG LI, MD
Department of Surgery, Competence Center of
Thoracic Surgery, Charité University Hospital
Berlin, Berlin, Germany

MARCO MAMMANA, MD
Thoracic Surgery Unit, Department
of Cardiologic, Thoracic and Vascular
Sciences, University Hospital, Padova,
Italy

GIUSEPPE MARULLI, MD, PhD
Thoracic Surgery Unit, Department of
Emergency and Organ Transplantation,
University Hospital, Bari, Italy

ANDREAS MEISEL, MD, PhD
Department of Neurology Berlin, Charité
University Hospital Berlin, Berlin, Germany

WENTAO MI, MD, PhD
Fellow, Department of Neurology, Jacobs
School of Medicine and Biomedical Sciences,
University at Buffalo/SUNY, Buffalo, New York,
USA

TOMMASO CLAUDIO MINEO, MD
Department of Surgery and Experimental
Medicine, Myasthenia Gravis Multidisciplinary
Program, Tor Vergata University, Rome,
Italy

LOULWAH MUKHARESH, MD
Chief Resident, Department of Neurology,
George Washington University, Washington,
DC, USA

GIUSEPPE NATALE, MD
Thoracic Surgery Unit, Department of
Cardiologic, Thoracic and Vascular Sciences,
University Hospital, Padova, Italy

FEDERICO REA, MD
Thoracic Surgery Unit, Department of
Cardiologic, Thoracic and Vascular Sciences,
University Hospital, Padova, Italy

JENS-C. RUECKERT, MD, PhD
Department of Surgery, Competence Center of
Thoracic Surgery, Charité University Hospital
Berlin, Berlin, Germany

MARCO SCHIAVON, MD, PhD
Thoracic Surgery Unit, Department of
Cardiologic, Thoracic and Vascular Sciences,
University Hospital, Padova, Italy

JOSEPH B. SHRAGER, MD
Professor and Chief, Division of Thoracic
Surgery, Department of Cardiothoracic
Surgery, Stanford University Hospitals and
Clinics, Stanford University School of
Medicine, Stanford, California, USA

NICHOLAS J. SILVESTRI, MD
Associate Professor, Department of
Neurology, Jacobs School of Medicine and
Biomedical Sciences, University at Buffalo/
SUNY, Buffalo, New York, USA

PUSPA THAPA, PhD
Postdoctoral Research Scientist, Columbia
Center for Translational Immunology,
Columbia University Irving Medical Center,
New York, New York, USA

DENIZ ULUK, MD
Department of Surgery, Competence Center of
Thoracic Surgery, Charité University Hospital
Berlin, Berlin, Germany

SEAN C. WIGHTMAN, MD
Division of Thoracic Surgery, Department of
Cardiothoracic Surgery, Stanford University
Hospitals and Clinics, Stanford University
School of Medicine, Stanford, California, USA

GIL I. WOLFE, MD
Irvin and Rosemary Smith Professor and
Chairman, University at Buffalo Distinguished
Professor, Department of Neurology, Jacobs
School of Medicine and Biomedical Sciences,
University at Buffalo/SUNY, Buffalo, New York,
USA

MARCIN ZIELIŃSKI, MD, PhD
Department of Thoracic Surgery, Pulmonary
Hospital, Ul. Gładkie 1, Zakopane, Poland

Contents

The Role of the Thymus in the Immune Response

Puspa Thapa and Donna L. Farber

The thymus is a primary lymphoid organ essential for the development of T lymphocytes, which orchestrate adaptive immune responses. T-cell development in the thymus is spatially regulated; key checkpoints in T-cell maturation and selection occur in cortical and medullary regions to eliminate self-reactive T cells, establish central tolerance, and export naïve T cells to the periphery with the potential to recognize diverse pathogens. Thymic output is also temporally regulated due to age-related involution of the thymus accompanied by loss of epithelial cells. This review discusses the structural and age-related control of thymus function in humans.

A Neurologist's Perspective on Understanding Myasthenia Gravis: Clinical Perspectives of Etiologic Factors, Diagnosis, and Preoperative Treatment

Loulwah Mukharesh and Henry J. Kaminski

Myasthenia gravis (MG) is a disease of neuromuscular transmission caused by antibodies directed toward proteins concentrated at the neuromuscular junction. Mild to life-threatening weakness varies in severity over time and with level of activity. Therefore, clinical diagnosis is often challenging. MG may be categorized by autoantibody type, thymic pathologic condition, and age of onset. Treatments are tailored for each group. A key management concern is severe exacerbation of weakness resulting from infections or exposure to certain medications, including antibiotics, which may be severe enough to produce respiratory decompensation. The article reviews key diagnostic issues and treatment options.

A Neurologist's Perspective on Thymectomy for Myasthenia Gravis: Current Perspective and Future Trials

Wentao Mi, Nicholas J. Silvestri, and Gil I. Wolfe

The first randomized blinded study of thymectomy in nonthymomatous myasthenia gravis was designed to answer 3 questions: does the combination of prednisone and removal of the thymus gland via extended transsternal thymectomy after 3 years compared with an identical dosing protocol of prednisone alone (1) lead to better disease status for generalized MG patients with antiacetylcholine receptor antibodies, (2) reduce their prednisone requirements, and/or (3) reduce the side-effect burden from medications used to treat the disease? The study demonstrated that thymectomy confers these benefits for patients and sets the stage for inquiries into the benefits of less-invasive approaches to thymic resection.

History of Thymectomy for Myasthenia Gravis

Joel D. Cooper

In the early 1900s, chance observations of improved symptoms in several myasthenic patients undergoing thyroidectomy for goiters with concomitant resection of the adjacent thymus gland, first suggested a possible association between the thymus and

be achieved with various techniques. The uniportal video-assisted transcervical technique allows minimally invasive surgery with a low complication rate, a good cosmetic result, and a short length of recovery.

THORACIC SURGERY CLINICS

SERIES OF RELATED INTEREST

Surgical Clinics
http://www.surgical.theclinics.com
Surgical Oncology Clinics
http://www.surgonc.theclinics.com
Advances in Surgery
http://www.advancessurgery.com

THE CLINICS ARE AVAILABLE ONLINE!
Access your subscription at:
www.theclinics.com

Preface

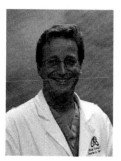

Joshua R. Sonett, MD
Editor

I am pleased to present this *Thoracic Surgery Clinics* dedicated to myasthenia gravis (MG) and thymectomy. The recent international prospectively randomized trial of thymectomy for MG (MGTX trial) has finally proven the effectiveness of thymectomy in nonthymomatous MG. The historical road to enable definitive proof of the role and effectiveness of thymectomy was led by many surgical leaders and thoracic surgical legends. We should be particularly indebted to Dr Fred Jaretzki, whose surgical leadership enabled the randomized international trial to come to fruition. The positive results of the trial, combined with the now many minimally invasive techniques to perform a thymectomy, should lead to a much wider acceptance and utilization of thymectomy in MG.

However, many unanswered questions remain in the treatment of this diverse population of patients, and early complete cure of this autoimmune disease remains elusive. Future progress and trials working toward maximizing the cure and treatment of these patients will need to be led by the next generation of thoracic surgeons. Understanding the immunologic role of the thymus, the current medical approach to the treatment of myasthenic patients, as well as the historical perspective of how we arrived at our current state of knowledge will be the key to the next developmental steps and progress toward cure.

I am blessed and grateful to have had so many leaders and experts in the field contribute to this issue of *Thoracic Surgery Clinics*. Each article was written by prominent respected physicians in the fields of immunology, neurology, and surgery. Given the many unanswered questions that remain in the treatment of MG, I urge you to carefully read each article in order to gain the unique perspective of each of the authors. Understanding the immunologic function and maturation of the thymus is clearly essential in truly making progress in treating this disease, and surgeons must be fully cognizant of these concepts in order to effectively integrate treatment in a multidisciplinary approach. Collaboration with our colleagues in neurology is essential to current treatment algorithms and future studies to improve outcomes in this disease. Finally, several surgical approaches are presented by surgeon champions of those techniques, offering valuable lessons regardless of one's personal bias.

I hope you enjoy reading these thoughtful articles as much as I did.

Joshua R. Sonett, MD
Columbia University Medical Center
New York-Presbyterian Hospital
Herbert Irving Pavilion
161 Fort Washington Avenue
3rd Floor
New York, NY 10032, USA

E-mail address:
js2106@cumc.columbia.edu

Thorac Surg Clin 29 (2019) ix
https://doi.org/10.1016/j.thorsurg.2019.02.001
1547-4127/19/© 2019 Published by Elsevier Inc.

The Role of the Thymus in the Immune Response

Puspa Thapa, PhD[a], Donna L. Farber, PhD[b],*

KEYWORDS

• T lymphocytes • Epithelial cells • Immunosenescence • T-cell development

KEY POINTS

• The thymus is a specialized organ that directs the development and selection of T cells, which direct adaptive immunity.
• Thymic function is spatially and temporally regulated and wanes with age.
• Thymic output is essential during early life to establish immune competence and homeostasis but is dispensable thereafter.

INTRODUCTION

The thymus is an organ that is critically important to the immune system, which serves as the body's defense mechanism, providing surveillance and protection against diverse pathogens, tumors, antigens, and mediators of tissue damage. The immune system comprises a complex network of cellular and molecular components subdivided into thymus-independent (innate) and thymus-dependent (adaptive) arms, which function synergistically in all immune responses. Innate immunity constitutes the first line of defense and is mediated by innate immune cells, such as tissue macrophage, dendritic cells (DCs), and granulocytes, which elicit their effector function within minutes to hours after antigen exposure. Innate cells become activated via germline-encoded pattern recognition receptors, including Toll-like receptors and nucleotide oligomerization domain (NOD)-like receptors, which recognize invariant features of pathogens (pathogen-associated molecular patterns) and tissue damage (for a review, see Brubaker and colleagues[1]). Once activated, innate cells, such as macrophages and neutrophils, can effectively clear antigens via phagocytosis. Other types of innate cells, such as DCs, take up and process antigens, resulting in expression of antigenic epitopes in conjunction with their major histocompatibility complex (MHC) or HLA molecules. These DCs can then serve as antigen-presenting cells for the priming of the adaptive immune system. In this way, the early innate response is coupled to and facilitates adaptive immunity.

The adaptive immune system consists of T lymphocytes and B lymphocytes, which express specific antigen recognition receptors and develop highly specialized effector functions with the ability to form long-term immunologic memory. Both B cells and T cells develop from bone marrow–derived progenitors; whereas mature B cells are exported to the periphery directly from the bone marrow, T-cell development, maturation, and export require critical differentiation steps to occur in the thymus. Thymus-dependent T-cell differentiation processes include expression of an antigen-specific cell surface T-cell receptor (TCR) through recombination of germline-encoded gene segments and thymic education involving negative selection of potentially self-reactive T cells and positive selection of T cells with the capacity to recognize antigens encountered in the

Disclosure Statement: NIH UOIAI100119.

[a] Columbia Center for Translational Immunology, Columbia University Medical Center, 650 West 168th Street, BB1501, New York, NY 10032, USA; [b] Department of Surgery, Columbia Center for Translational Immunology, Columbia University Medical Center, 650 West 168th Street, BB1501, New York, NY 10032, USA
* Corresponding author.
E-mail address: df2396@cumc.columbia.edu

Thorac Surg Clin 29 (2019) 123–131
https://doi.org/10.1016/j.thorsurg.2018.12.001
1547-4127/19/

periphery. These important thymic processes ensure that T cells can recognize antigens in the context of self-MHC but do not elicit self-reactivity.

Once exported from the thymus, the resultant naïve T cells populate multiple secondary lymphoid organs, including spleen and many lymph nodes. Naïve T cells become activated by antigens presented by DCs in lymphoid sites, resulting in T-cell proliferation and differentiation to effector cells, which can migrate to diverse tissues sites of pathogen encounter. Different types of effector T cells mediate diverse functions, including enhancing inflammatory responses, mediating direct cellular cytotoxicity against virally infected cells or tumor cells or helping B cells differentiate to antibody-secreting cells, and class switching of different antibody isotypes. A majority of antibody responses to protein antigens and viral and bacterial pathogens require T-cell help; however, there are 2 types of B cell-responses that occur independent of T cells. Certain types of antigens, such as repeating polysaccharides within bacterial cell walls, can directly cross-link the B-cell antigen receptor and activate B cells and have been referred to as thymus-independent antigens. In addition, natural antibodies that form part of the innate immune also can be generated in the absence of T cells.[2] Aside from these exceptions, T cells are essential for most aspects of adaptive immunity, and, because the innate immune response itself cannot effectively clear most pathogens, life without T cells is not sustainable.

The role of the thymus in the development and function of T cells is a highly regulated process within the tissue; specific differentiation and events occur in cortical and medullary regions[3] and are regulated with age. The thymus structure comprises specialized stromal cells, designated thymic epithelial cells (TECs), consisting of 2 major subsets, cortical TECs (cTECs) and medullary TECs (mTECs), that govern both positive and negative selection of T cells; the localization and interaction of developing thymocytes with TEC subsets is critical for proper T-cell export.[4] In addition, thymic output is also highly regulated by age and life stage; thymic-dependent production of T cells is critical during fetal development and early life but is dispensable thereafter and wanes during early adulthood. Infants born lacking proper development of a thymus (due to DiGeorge syndrome or FoxN1 mutations) suffer from life-threatening infections, resulting in early mortality during the first year of life due to reduced numbers and impaired function of peripheral T cells.[5–7] Thymus transplantation during early life can establish normal T-cell numbers and function and enable these individuals to survive and thrive.[5,6,8] By contrast,

thymectomy during infancy and early childhood typically is performed during cardiac surgery for repair of congenital abnormalities and does not compromise peripheral T-cell functions and immune responses,[9,10] because infants are born with a full T-cell complement in the periphery. In addition, there are multiple peripheral mechanisms for maintaining T-cell numbers, which have been partly elucidated in mice and are just beginning to be understood in humans.

This review discusses how the complex structure of thymus provides a unique microenvironment to orchestrate the differentiation of thymocytes and TEC and educates T cells to recognize self from nonself. How T-cell development occurs in the thymus and the developmental checkpoints that thymocytes progress through to become mature T cells exported to the periphery are reviewed. Age-related regulation of thymic function based on results from mouse and human studies and implications for immunosenescence and regulation also are discussed.

THYMIC STRUCTURE AND DEVELOPMENT

The development of TECs is critical for thymic organogenesis, which occurs during fetal development. Studies using mouse embryos have elucidated several factors intrinsic to TECs that play crucial roles in the development of thymic structure both prenatally and postnatally.[3,11] The transcription factor FoxN1 is critical for all TEC development and maintenance (fetal and postnatal); loss of FoxN1 leads to loss of thymic structure and autoimmune disease in both humans and mice.[12–17] FoxN1 is highly expressed by embryonic TECs and at least 50% of postnatal TECs retain FoxN1 expression, highlighting its importance.[18] The regulation of FoxN1 expression in TEC is not fully understood although signaling pathways, such as the bone morphogenetic protein and wingless/integrated factors, have been described.[19,20] Considerably less is known about the regulation of FoxN1 in humans and its role in maintaining thymus integrity.

The proper development of thymus tissue requires the generation of structurally and functionally distinct cortical and medullary regions via development of cTECs and mTECs, respectively. Early fetal TECs are bipotent, giving rise to both cortical and medullary epithelial cells (cTECs and mTECs, respectively).[12,21,22] After homing to the thymic structure, the differentiation of cTECs and mTECs is perpetuated by additional mechanisms unique to each cortical or medullary epithelial cell lineage. The cTEC and mTEC lineages exhibit distinct expression of specific markers; cTECs can be identified by surface expression of cytokeratin 8, Ly51, and CD205 whereas mTECs express cytokeratin 5, CD80, and UEA1.[23] Although these markers identify the specific TEC lineage, expression of these factors varies within each subset, which may reflect maturation stages.[3,24] Recent studies on transcriptome profiling of murine TECs on the single-cell level revealed that cellular heterogeneity of TECs may be reflection of the developmental stage of TECs.[25]

Another key transcription factor important in TEC function, designated autoimmune regulator (AIRE) protein is specifically expressed by mTECs and functions to induce promiscuous expression of tissue-restricted antigens (TRAs), such as insulin (pancreas-specific) and kidney-specific proteins.[26–31] The presentation of TRA by mTECS is one of the key mechanisms that leads to deletion of self-reactive or autoreactive T cells in the thymus establishing central tolerance. *AIRE* deficiency leads to robust autoimmunity in both humans and mice.[32,33] In humans, AIRE dysfunction leads to a rare disorder called autoimmune polyendocrinopathy-candidiasis-ectodermal dystrophy,[26] characterized by multiendocrine autoimmune disease, chronic mucocutaneous candidiasis, and dystrophy of dental enamel and nails.[34] More than 40 mutations in the *AIRE* gene that leads to dysfunctional protein have been identified to cause this autosomal recessive inherited disease.[34] Together, the TEC-specific factors not only are crucial for thymic structural integrity but also play key roles in the promoting the development and selection of thymocytes, as described later.

T-CELL DEVELOPMENT IN THE THYMUS

The earliest stage for T-cell development originates in the bone marrow as hematopoietic stem cells, which are self-renewing and can differentiate into both myeloid and lymphoid progenitors; the latter give rise to both T lymphocytes and B lymphocytes. Lymphoid progenitors circulate out of the bone marrow and those expressing platelet (P)-selected glycoprotein ligand 1 (PSGL1) enter the thymus via their interaction with P-selectin on thymic endothelial cells. Additional thymus homing signals are received via chemokines binding to CCR7 and CCR9 on the progenitor cells.[35–37] This thymus homing step is the earliest step in the development of functional T cells, described later and diagrammed in **Fig. 1**.

The migration of thymocytes within the thymic microenvironment directs their proper development.[38,39] Thymocytes are guided by various chemokines secreted by stromal cells, including cTECS and mTECs that govern their movement from medullary to the cortical region and back to medullary region within the thymus before egress to the periphery (see **Fig. 1**). Beginning in the cortical-medullary junction, bone marrow–derived lymphoid progenitors first commit to the T-cell lineage by receiving notch ligands (DLL4) and interleukin (IL)-7 provided by cTECs to become early thymic precursors (ETPs),[40,41] also designated as double-negative (DN) thymocytes for their lack of expression of CD4 and CD8 coreceptors, which are markers of mature T cells. DN1/ETPs proceed on to migrate toward the subcapsular cortical region, triggering their development into DN2 and DN3 stages where they begin to rearrange the *TRB* locus,[42,43] and express CD25/CD44 (see **Fig. 1**). Maturation to the DN3 stage involves a β-selection checkpoint where thymocytes progress onto the next developmental stage only when they are successful in generating an inframe TCRβ chain rearrangement. The rearranged TCRβ chain is paired with a pre-TCRα chain and tested for its ability to form a cell surface pre-TCR complex.[44] Successful expression of the pre-TCR complex initiates the proliferation and differentiation from DN3 to DN4 and to double-positive (DP) (CD4$^+$CD8$^+$) thymocytes characterized by coexpression of both coreceptors.[45,46] These DP cells form the majority of thymocytes in the thymus during early life.[47]

Formation of DP thymocytes is a key step in T-cell development, because it is this stage that undergoes final maturation and selection for potential export to the periphery. The mature TCR complex is formed during this DP stage after *TRA* rearrangement, expression of a functional TCRα chain, and association with the TCRβ chain and CD3 signaling molecules. DP thymocytes expressing mature TCRs subsequently undergo positive selection for recognition of peptides in the context of self-MHC. Through this process, low avidity recognition of self-peptide:self-MHC on cTECs by the TCR complex leads to a positive signal for survival (such as Bcl-2) whereas no recognition leads to death by neglect.[48] The recognition of self-peptide:self-MHC is also in part governed by the coreceptors CD4 and CD8-promoting lineage choice to be single-positive (SP) cells expressing either the CD4 or CD8 coreceptor[49] (see **Fig. 1**). These newly generated SP T cells are still not ready for export, because they require another selection event to screen for self-reactive T cells.

After positive selection, SP T cells increase their expression of CCR7 and migrate to the medullary region via CCL19 and CCL21 produced by mTECs.[42,43] In the medulla, SP CD4$^+$ and SP CD8$^+$ T cells undergo a process called negative

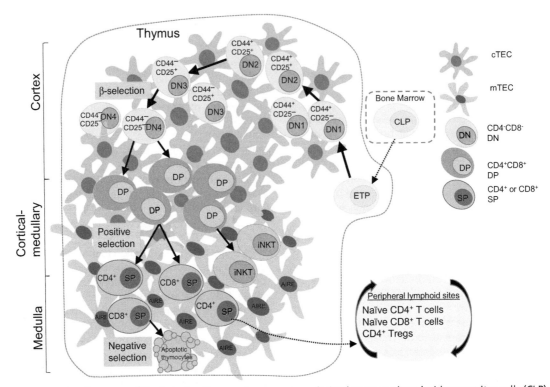

Fig. 1. The development of T cells in the thymus. Bone marrow–derived common lymphoid progenitor cells (CLP) enter the thymus to begin commitment to the T-cell lineage as early thymic precursors (ETP). ETPs differentiate to DN thymocytes (*tan–orange*), based on the lack of expression of CD4 and CD8 coreceptors. DN thymocytes progress through sequential DN1–4 stages, as defined by the coordinate expression of CD44 and CD25 on the cell surface. The TCRβ chain is expressed at DN3, triggering progression and maturation to DP thymocytes (*pink*), expressing both CD4 and CD8 coreceptors. Positive selection delineates selection of thymocytes into the CD4, T-helper, or CD8 cytotoxic T-cell lineage to become SP CD4 or SP CD8 T cells (*maroon*). After positive selection, SP CD4[+] or SP CD8[+] T cells migrate to the medulla to go through negative selection mediated by mTECs, where autoreactive SP T cells are deleted by apoptosis, whereas SP T cells that pass negative selection are exported to the periphery. This process of thymopoiesis results in population of peripheral blood and lymphoid sites with naïve CD4[+] and CD8[+] T cells and CD4 Tregs.

selection, whereby self-reactive T cells are deleted, establishing central tolerance. During negative selection, SP T cells are presented TRAs by mTECs and tested for their affinity toward self-antigen.[29] Strong recognition of self-peptide leads to apoptosis mediated by Bim proapoptotic molecule and deletion of self-reactive T cells before they can migrate to the periphery and potentially trigger autoimmunity.[50,51] Together, these studies show that the thymic structure is highly organized, with distinct cortical and medullary compartments to facilitate the proper development and selection of T cells with the ability to protect but not generate self-reactivity.

The thymic selection events, described previously, are stringent; a majority (>95%) of developing T cells fail positive or negative selection and die or fail to be exported. A full complement of naïve CD4[+] and CD8[+] T cells emerges, however, after this rigorous selection, which collectively express a diverse array of TCRs with the potential to recognize millions of different antigenic epitopes. Naïve CD4[+] T cells recognizing epitopes presented by MHC class II molecules can be activated and differentiate to T-helper effector cells for coordinating all aspects of cellular immunity to diverse pathogens; naïve CD8[+] T cells recognizing epitopes presented by MHC class I molecules differentiate into cytotoxic T cells important for antiviral and antitumor immunity. A third type of T-cell lineage, designated regulatory T cells (Tregs), also develops in the thymus as a result of the same selection events. Tregs are distinguished by their expression of the Foxp3 transcription factor and are required in the periphery for proper immunoregulation and prevention of autoimmunity.[52] Tregs experience stronger positive selection signals and are more self-reactive than other conventional T cells[53] and, therefore, result from a third decision point in the selection process. Tregs also express diverse TCRs but are distinct from TCRs expressed by conventional naïve CD4$^+$ T-cell counterparts.[54]

In addition to mature T cells with diverse TCRs, a type of innate-like T cells, called natural killer T (NKT) cells, also develop in the thymus. NKT cells are designated as innate T cells because they respond rapidly (minutes to hours) after stimulation and exhibit a limited TCR repertoire (and therefore limited specificity) with a majority of NKT cells expressing a common alpha chain, Vα24 in human and Vα14 in mice paired with Jα18.[55] NKT cells also undergo positive selection at the DP thymocytes stage in the thymus but are selected by other DP thymocytes presenting endogenous glycolipids on CD1d molecules. NKT cells experience stronger TCR signal during positive selection and express PLZF, a transcriptional factor that commits NKT cells to their lineage.[53,56] Although NKT cells share a common progenitor stage (DP) as conventional T cells, they have distinct transcriptional programs that direct their commitment to NKT cells on positive selection.[57,58] Several transcription factors have been identified that regulate the positive selection of NKT cells but not conventional T cells at the DP thymocyte stage.[57] NKT cells have diverse effector functions with cytotoxic capacity and both proinflammatory and anti-inflammatory cytokine production and are potential targets for immunotherapies in cancer and autoimmunity.[59] The thymus, therefore, serves a key role in promoting and directing the development and selection of multiple types of T lymphocytes, with specific functional roles in immune responses.

THYMIC INVOLUTION AND AGING

Much of the knowledge about thymus integrity and thymopoiesis derives from studies in mice, which have been essential in revealing the molecular mechanisms underlying these processes. Human studies have provided new insights into the key differences between mice and humans in this regard. Mice are born lymphopenic and have a small thymus that grows in size before it involutes with age. Unlike mice, humans are born with a full complement of T cells in circulation and lymphoid tissues, and the human thymus is largest at birth and is most active up until puberty. After puberty, the thymus starts to involute with age and turns into fatty tissue.[60] The timing requirement for thymic output in immunoregulation also differs in mice and humans. Neonatal thymectomy in mice can give rise to lethal autoimmunity marked by multiorgan infiltrates, which has been shown to occur due to a lack of Treg maturation.[61,62] By

contrast, neonatal thymectomy in humans that has been performed during infant cardiac surgery is not associated with autoimmunity later in life, and individuals develop and maintain normal frequencies of Tregs in peripheral blood.[63,64] Similarly, individuals who experienced neonatal thymectomy (and are now in their third to fourth decades of life) do not exhibit increased susceptibility to infections during the critical window of childhood.[65] Together, these results indicate that the certain key events in thymus-dependent T-cell development and the contribution of thymic output to establishing T-cell homeostasis is largely set prenatally and during the early postnatal period in humans.

Despite the lack of overt immune dysregulation within individuals thymectomized in early life, there are several caveats that should be taken into consideration in evaluating these data. First, mediastinal extraction of the thymus during cardiac surgery may not remove all thymus tissue, because thymic remnants may extend into cervical regions[66,67] and could mediate partial thymic function. In addition, the peripheral T-cell compartment, including T-cell numbers early after thymectomy and the proportion of naïve and memory T cells, is altered in thymectomized individuals compared with individuals with an intact thymus. There is an early reduction in T-cell numbers after thymectomy and several studies have reported an accelerated accumulation of memory T cells in thymectomized compared with control individuals,[10,68–70] indicating that thymic output later in life is important for replenishing naïve T cells and maintaining the ability to respond to new pathogens. Thymectomized populations are living in the modern era, with advanced hygiene and low pathogen load, and also have generally received childhood vaccinations. Therefore, the lack of naïve T cells later in life may not have the same consequences in an environment of high pathogen load.

During normal human aging, the thymus continues its active process of thymopoiesis into the fourth decade of life, manifested by the presence of active thymic tissue with DP thymocytes, which are greatly reduced after 40 years of age.[71] Thymic output also can be measured by assessing the presence of TCR excision circles in naïve T cells marking recent thymic emigrants in both mice and human.[72] These studies show that with age, the presence of TCR excision circles also declines, with a precipitous decrease after age 40, indicating lower thymic output in humans.[73,74] In contrast, mice at 2 years of age are fully capable of generating recent thymic emigrants, indicating that mice thymic output is independent of age-related thymic size.[75] Direct comparison studies showed that in humans the naïve T-cell compartment is largely maintained by homeostatic turnover in the periphery and not by thymic output whereas thymic output maintains T cells numbers throughout the much shorter mouse lifetime.[72] These peripheral mechanisms involve the action of homeostatic and T-cell survival cytokines, such as IL-7 and IL-15, and contact of T cells with cognate or noncognate stimuli, as defined in mouse models. In humans, the molecular mechanisms underlying peripheral T-cell turnover have not been elucidated; however, recent evidence suggests that lymph nodes may create a tissue reservoir for long-term maintenance of naïve and resting T cells.[71,76]

The thymus atrophies with age in both mice and humans; however, mechanisms driving thymic involution are still not fully understood.[77,78] In mouse models and humans, the loss of TECs seems associated primarily with thymic atrophy and reductions in thymopoiesis, with several factors playing important roles in this process. The expression of the key TEC transcription factor, FoxN1, decreases with age, causing rapid degradation of TECs, whereas forced expressed of FoxN1 reversed thymic degradation.[13,17] Moreover, expression of thymopoeisis-promoting factors, such as IL-7 and MHC Class II, is also reduced in TECs with age.[79–81] Loss of either factor inhibits the ability of TECs to interact and provide growth factors to developing thymocytes, thereby inhibiting thymopoiesis. With increasing age, TECs do not readily regenerate, leading to hypostromal structure and enabling fat cells to accumulate and fill the thymic space in humans.[82,83] Cell ablation studies in mouse models suggest that cTEC may exhibit regeneration capacities during aging,[84] suggesting that therapeutic targeting of this subset could be a promising area for boosting thymic activity.

Sex hormones may also play an important role in thymic regeneration. Thymic involution occurs at a faster rate in male mice compared to female mice, suggesting a role for androgens in thymic atrophy.[85,86] Consistent with this idea, gonadal steroid hormones have been shown to have a negative on impact TEC survival, and conversely, sex steroid ablation therapy leads to an increase in thymus size and thymocyte development.[85,87,88] Together, the reduction in epithelial cell turnover and expression of key TEC-associated transcription factors coupled with age-related and gender-related effects on thymic structural integrity and increased fat accumulation result in reduced homing of bone marrow progenitors and induction of thymopoiesis.

CONCLUSION

The thymus provides a specialized microenvironment for the development of highly diverse and functional T cells that are also tolerant to self. Thymopoiesis is spatially regulated within the thymus, with distinct checkpoints occurring as thymocytes progress through their developmental stages from the cortical-medullary region to the cortex, where cTECs mediate positive selection. On positive selection, SP thymocytes migrate to the medulla, where mTECs govern negative selection to delete autoreactive T cells, establishing central tolerance. Thymopoiesis results in a full complement of peripheral naïve T cells with diverse recognition capacity against diverse pathogens and subsets of Tregs to inhibit overactive immune responses and autoimmunity. This highly regulated process is quite active at birth in humans; however, thymic involution associated with reduced TEC content and integrity begins during early childhood and continues through adulthood, resulting in a loss of thymic structural integrity and cessation of thymopoiesis that occurs well before the natural end of the human life span. Remarkably, much of the functional and regulatory aspects of thymus-dependent T-cell responses occur early in life and may be largely dispensable thereafter; multiple peripheral mechanisms for homeostasis maintain T-cell numbers and proper immunoregulation. Targeting thymic regeneration and modulation of thymic output nevertheless can be therapeutic for boosting production of new naïve T cells in vaccines and promoting human T-cell reconstitution after treatments that severely depletes T cells, such as in bone marrow transplantation and chemotherapy and after severe viral infections. A greater understanding of these processes in human thymic tissue will be important for translating findings from mice to humans and revealing mechanisms underlying the complexity of the human thymus.

REFERENCES

1. Brubaker SW, Bonham KS, Zanoni I, et al. Innate immune pattern recognition: a cell biological perspective. Annu Rev Immunol 2015;33(1):257–90.
2. Kaveri SV, Silverman GJ, Bayry J. Natural IgM in immune equilibrium and harnessing their therapeutic potential. J Immunol 2012;188(3):939–45.
3. Takahama Y, Ohigashi I, Baik S, et al. Generation of diversity in thymic epithelial cells. Nat Rev Immunol 2017;17(5):295–305.
4. Shores EW, Van Ewijk W, Singer A. Disorganization and restoration of thymic medullary epithelial cells in T cell receptor-negative scid mice: evidence that

receptor-bearing lymphocytes influence maturation of the thymic microenvironment. Eur J Immunol 1991;21(7):1657–61.

5. Markert ML, Sarzotti M, Ozaki DA, et al. Thymus transplantation in complete DiGeorge syndrome: immunologic and safety evaluations in 12 patients. Blood 2003;102(3):1121–30.

6. Chinn IK, Milner JD, Scheinberg P, et al. Thymus transplantation restores the repertoires of forkhead box protein 3 (FoxP3)+ and FoxP3- T cells in complete DiGeorge anomaly. Clin Exp Immunol 2013; 173(1):140–9.

7. Amorosi S, D'Armiento M, Calcagno G, et al. FOXN1 homozygous mutation associated with anencephaly and severe neural tube defect in human athymic Nude/SCID fetus. Clin Genet 2008;73(4):380–4.

8. Markert ML, Marques JG, Neven B, et al. First use of thymus transplantation therapy for FOXN1 deficiency (nude/SCID): a report of 2 cases. Blood 2011;117(2):688–96.

9. Roosen J, Oosterlinck W, Meyns B. Routine thymectomy in congenital cardiac surgery changes adaptive immunity without clinical relevance. Interact Cardiovasc Thorac Surg 2015;20(1):101–6.

10. Sauce D, Appay V. Altered thymic activity in early life: how does it affect the immune system in young adults? Curr Opin Immunol 2011;23(4):543–8.

11. Abramson J, Anderson G. Thymic epithelial cells. Annu Rev Immunol 2017;35:85–118.

12. Bleul CC, Corbeaux T, Reuter A, et al. Formation of a functional thymus initiated by a postnatal epithelial progenitor cell. Nature 2006;441(7096):992–6.

13. Chen L, Xiao S, Manley NR. Foxn1 is required to maintain the postnatal thymic microenvironment in a dosage-sensitive manner. Blood 2009;113(3): 567–74.

14. Corbeaux T, Hess I, Swann JB, et al. Thymopoiesis in mice depends on a Foxn1-positive thymic epithelial cell lineage. Proc Natl Acad Sci U S A 2010; 107(38):16613–8.

15. Cheng L, Guo J, Sun L, et al. Postnatal tissue-specific disruption of transcription factor FoxN1 triggers acute thymic atrophy. J Biol Chem 2010;285(8): 5836–47.

16. Zuklys S, Handel A, Zhanybekova S, et al. Foxn1 regulates key target genes essential for T cell development in postnatal thymic epithelial cells. Nat Immunol 2016;17(10):1206–15.

17. Xu M, Sizova O, Wang L, et al. A fine-tune role of Mir-125a-5p on Foxn1 during age-associated changes in the thymus. Aging Dis 2017;8(3):277–86.

18. Rode I, Martins VC, Kublbeck G, et al. Foxn1 protein expression in the developing, aging, and regenerating thymus. J Immunol 2015;195(12):5678–87.

19. Bleul CC, Boehm T. BMP signaling is required for normal thymus development. J Immunol 2005; 175(8):5213–21.

20. Balciunaite G, Keller MP, Balciunaite E, et al. Wnt glycoproteins regulate the expression of FoxN1, the gene defective in nude mice. Nat Immunol 2002;3(11):1102–8.

21. Kingston R, Jenkinson EJ, Owen JJ. A single stem cell can recolonize an embryonic thymus, producing phenotypically distinct T-cell populations. Nature 1985;317(6040):811–3.

22. Rodewald HR, Paul S, Haller C, et al. Thymus medulla consisting of epithelial islets each derived from a single progenitor. Nature 2001;414(6865): 763–8.

23. Rossi SW, Jeker LT, Ueno T, et al. Keratinocyte growth factor (KGF) enhances postnatal T-cell development via enhancements in proliferation and function of thymic epithelial cells. Blood 2007; 109(9):3803–11.

24. Alexandropoulos K, Danzl NM. Thymic epithelial cells: antigen presenting cells that regulate T cell repertoire and tolerance development. Immunol Res 2012;54(1–3):177–90.

25. Kernfeld EM, Genga RMJ, Neherin K, et al. A single-cell transcriptomic atlas of thymus organogenesis resolves cell types and developmental maturation. Immunity 2018;48(6):1258–70.e6.

26. Liston A, Gray DH, Lesage S, et al. Gene dosage-limiting role of Aire in thymic expression, clonal deletion, and organ-specific autoimmunity. J Exp Med 2004;200(8):1015–26.

27. Anderson MS, Venanzi ES, Chen Z, et al. The cellular mechanism of Aire control of T cell tolerance. Immunity 2005;23(2):227–39.

28. Gray D, Abramson J, Benoist C, et al. Proliferative arrest and rapid turnover of thymic epithelial cells expressing Aire. J Exp Med 2007;204(11):2521–8.

29. Irla M, Hugues S, Gill J, et al. Autoantigen-specific interactions with CD4+ thymocytes control mature medullary thymic epithelial cell cellularity. Immunity 2008;29(3):451–63.

30. Hansenne I, Louis C, Martens H, et al. Aire and Foxp3 expression in a particular microenvironment for T cell differentiation. Neuroimmunomodulation 2009;16(1):35–44.

31. Liston A, Lesage S, Wilson J, et al. Aire regulates negative selection of organ-specific T cells. Nat Immunol 2003;4(4):350–4.

32. Kisand K, Peterson P. Autoimmune polyendocrinopathy candidiasis ectodermal dystrophy: known and novel aspects of the syndrome. Ann N Y Acad Sci 2011;1246:77–91.

33. Peterson P, Org T, Rebane A. Transcriptional regulation by AIRE: molecular mechanisms of central tolerance. Nat Rev Immunol 2008;8(12):948–57.

34. Ahonen P, Myllärniemi S, Sipilä I, et al. Clinical variation of autoimmune polyendocrinopathy–candidiasis–ectodermal dystrophy (APECED) in a series of 68 patients. N Engl J Med 1990;322(26):1829–36.

35. Rossi FM, Corbel SY, Merzaban JS, et al. Recruitment of adult thymic progenitors is regulated by P-selectin and its ligand PSGL-1. Nat Immunol 2005; 6(6):626–34.

36. Krueger A, Willenzon S, Lyszkiewicz M, et al. CC chemokine receptor 7 and 9 double-deficient hematopoietic progenitors are severely impaired in seeding the adult thymus. Blood 2010;115(10): 1906–12.

37. Zlotoff DA, Sambandam A, Logan TD, et al. CCR7 and CCR9 together recruit hematopoietic progenitors to the adult thymus. Blood 2010;115(10): 1897–905.

38. Lind EF, Prockop SE, Porritt HE, et al. Mapping precursor movement through the postnatal thymus reveals specific microenvironments supporting defined stages of early lymphoid development. J Exp Med 2001;194(2):127–34.

39. Takahama Y. Journey through the thymus: stromal guides for T-cell development and selection. Nat Rev Immunol 2006;6(2):127–35.

40. Radtke F, Wilson A, Stark G, et al. Deficient T cell fate specification in mice with an induced inactivation of Notch1. Immunity 1999;10(5):547–58.

41. Peschon JJ, Morrissey PJ, Grabstein KH, et al. Early lymphocyte expansion is severely impaired in interleukin 7 receptor-deficient mice. J Exp Med 1994; 180(5):1955–60.

42. Ueno T, Saito F, Gray DH, et al. CCR7 signals are essential for cortex-medulla migration of developing thymocytes. J Exp Med 2004;200(4):493–505.

43. Kurobe H, Liu C, Ueno T, et al. CCR7-dependent cortex-to-medulla migration of positively selected thymocytes is essential for establishing central tolerance. Immunity 2006;24(2):165–77.

44. Krangel MS. Mechanics of T cell receptor gene rearrangement. Curr Opin Immunol 2009;21(2): 133–9.

45. Gascoigne NRJ, Rybakin V, Acuto O, et al. TCR signal strength and T cell development. Annu Rev Cell Dev Biol 2016;32(1):327–48.

46. Fehling HJ, Krotkova A, Saint-Ruf C, et al. Crucial role of the pre-T-cell receptor alpha gene in development of alpha beta but not gamma delta T cells. Nature 1995;375(6534):795–8.

47. Cuddihy AR, Ge S, Zhu J, et al. VEGF-mediated cross-talk within the neonatal murine thymus. Blood 2009;113(12):2723.

48. McKean DJ, Huntoon CJ, Bell MP, et al. Maturation versus death of developing double-positive thymocytes reflects competing effects on Bcl-2 expression and can be regulated by the intensity of CD28 costimulation. J Immunol 2001;166(5):3468–75.

49. Bhandoola A, Cibotti R, Punt JA, et al. Positive selection as a developmental progression initiated by αβTCR signals that fix TCR specificity prior to lineage commitment. Immunity 1999;10(3):301–11.

50. Sohn SJ, Thompson J, Winoto A. Apoptosis during negative selection of autoreactive thymocytes. Curr Opin Immunol 2007;19(5):510–5.

51. Bouillet P, Purton JF, Godfrey DI, et al. BH3-only Bcl-2 family member Bim is required for apoptosis of autoreactive thymocytes. Nature 2002;415(6874):922–6.

52. Ziegler SF. FOXP3: of mice and men. Annu Rev Immunol 2006;24:209–26.

53. Moran AE, Holzapfel KL, Xing Y, et al. T cell receptor signal strength in Treg and iNKT cell development demonstrated by a novel fluorescent reporter mouse. J Exp Med 2011;208(6):1279–89.

54. Golding A, Darko S, Wylie WH, et al. Deep sequencing of the TCR-beta repertoire of human forkhead box protein 3 (FoxP3)(+) and FoxP3(-) T cells suggests that they are completely distinct and non-overlapping. Clin Exp Immunol 2017; 188(1):12–21.

55. Das R, Sant'Angelo DB, Nichols KE. Transcriptional control of invariant NKT cell development. Immunol Rev 2010;238(1):195–215.

56. Seiler MP, Mathew R, Liszewski MK, et al. Elevated and sustained expression of the transcription factors Egr1 and Egr2 controls NKT lineage differentiation in response to TCR signaling. Nat Immunol 2012;13(3): 264–71.

57. Thapa P, Das J, McWilliams D, et al. The transcriptional repressor NKAP is required for the development of iNKT cells. Nat Commun 2013;4:1582.

58. Kim EY, Lynch L, Brennan PJ, et al. The transcriptional programs of iNKT cells. Semin Immunol 2015;27(1):26–32.

59. Wu L, Gabriel CL, Parekh VV, et al. Invariant natural killer T cells: innate-like T cells with potent immunomodulatory activities. Tissue Antigens 2009;73(6): 535–45.

60. Haynes BF, Markert ML, Sempowski GD, et al. The role of the thymus in immune reconstitution in aging, bone marrow transplantation, and HIV-1 infection. Annu Rev Immunol 2000;18:529–60.

61. Asano M, Toda M, Sakaguchi N, et al. Autoimmune disease as a consequence of developmental abnormality of a T cell subpopulation. J Exp Med 1996; 184(2):387–96.

62. Sakaguchi S, Takahashi T, Nishizuka Y. Study on cellular events in postthymectomy autoimmune oophoritis in mice. I. Requirement of Lyt-1 effector cells for oocytes damage after adoptive transfer. J Exp Med 1982;156(6):1565–76.

63. Silva SL, Albuquerque AS, Serra-Caetano A, et al. Human naive regulatory T-cells feature high steady-state turnover and are maintained by IL-7. Oncotarget 2016;7(11):12163–75.

64. Silva SL, Albuquerque A, Amaral AJ, et al. Autoimmunity and allergy control in adults submitted to complete thymectomy early in infancy. PLoS One 2017;12(7):e0180385.

65. Mancebo E, Clemente J, Sanchez J, et al. Longitudinal analysis of immune function in the first 3 years of life in thymectomized neonates during cardiac surgery. Clin Exp Immunol 2008;154(3):375–83.

66. Yu L, Ma S, Jing Y, et al. Combined unilateral-thoracoscopic and mediastinoscopic thymectomy. Ann Thorac Surg 2010;90(6):2068–70.

67. Costa NS, Laor T, Donnelly LF. Superior cervical extension of the thymus; a normal finding that should not be mistaken for a mass. Radiology 2010;256(1): 238–42.

68. van den Broek T, Delemarre EM, Janssen WJ, et al. Neonatal thymectomy reveals differentiation and plasticity within human naive T cells. J Clin Invest 2016;126(3):1126–36.

69. Eysteinsdottir JH, Freysdottir J, Haraldsson A, et al. The influence of partial or total thymectomy during open heart surgery in infants on the immune function later in life. Clin Exp Immunol 2004;136(2):349–55.

70. Prelog M, Keller M, Geiger R, et al. Thymectomy in early childhood: significant alterations of the CD4(+)CD45RA(+)CD62L(+) T cell compartment in later life. Clin Immunol 2009;130(2):123–32.

71. Thome JJ, Grinshpun B, Kumar BV, et al. Longterm maintenance of human naive T cells through in situ homeostasis in lymphoid tissue sites. Sci Immunol 2016;1(6) [pii:eaah6506].

72. den Braber I, Mugwagwa T, Vrisekoop N, et al. Maintenance of peripheral naive T cells is sustained by thymus output in mice but not humans. Immunity 2012;36(2):288–97.

73. Nasi M, Troiano L, Lugli E, et al. Thymic output and functionality of the IL-7/IL-7 receptor system in centenarians: implications for the neolymphogenesis at the limit of human life. Aging Cell 2006;5(2):167–75.

74. Mitchell WA, Lang PO, Aspinall R. Tracing thymic output in older individuals. Clin Exp Immunol 2010; 161(3):497–503.

75. Hale JS, Boursalian TE, Turk GL, et al. Thymic output in aged mice. Proc Natl Acad Sci U S A 2006; 103(22):8447–52.

76. Miron M, Kumar BV, Meng W, et al. Human lymph nodes maintain TCF-1(hi) memory T cells with high functional potential and clonal diversity throughout life. J Immunol 2018;201(7):2132–40.

77. Lynch HE, Goldberg GL, Chidgey A, et al. Thymic involution and immune reconstitution. Trends Immunol 2009;30(7):366–73.

78. Palmer DB. The effect of age on thymic function. Front Immunol 2013;4:316.

79. Erickson M, Morkowski S, Lehar S, et al. Regulation of thymic epithelium by keratinocyte growth factor. Blood 2002;100(9):3269–78.

80. Zamisch M, Moore-Scott B, Su DM, et al. Ontogeny and regulation of IL-7-expressing thymic epithelial cells. J Immunol 2005;174(1):60–7.

81. Ribeiro AR, Rodrigues PM, Meireles C, et al. Thymocyte selection regulates the homeostasis of IL-7-expressing thymic cortical epithelial cells in vivo. J Immunol 2013;191(3):1200–9.

82. Yang H, Youm YH, Sun Y, et al. Axin expression in thymic stromal cells contributes to an age-related increase in thymic adiposity and is associated with reduced thymopoiesis independently of ghrelin signaling. J Leukoc Biol 2009;85(6):928–38.

83. Gruver AL, Hudson LL, Sempowski GD. Immunosenescence of ageing. J Pathol 2007;211(2):144–56.

84. Rode I, Boehm T. Regenerative capacity of adult cortical thymic epithelial cells. Proc Natl Acad Sci U S A 2012;109(9):3463–8.

85. Olsen NJ, Olson G, Viselli SM, et al. Androgen receptors in thymic epithelium modulate thymus size and thymocyte development. Endocrinology 2001; 142(3):1278–83.

86. Gui J, Morales AJ, Maxey SE, et al. MCL1 increases primitive thymocyte viability in female mice and promotes thymic expansion into adulthood. Int Immunol 2011;23(10):647–59.

87. Zoller AL, Kersh GJ. Estrogen induces thymic atrophy by eliminating early thymic progenitors and inhibiting proliferation of beta-selected thymocytes. J Immunol 2006;176(12):7371–8.

88. Sutherland JS, Goldberg GL, Hammett MV, et al. Activation of thymic regeneration in mice and humans following androgen blockade. J Immunol 2005;175(4):2741–53.

A Neurologist's Perspective on Understanding Myasthenia Gravis

Clinical Perspectives of Etiologic Factors, Diagnosis, and Preoperative Treatment

Loulwah Mukharesh, MD, Henry J. Kaminski, MD*

KEYWORDS

- Myasthenia gravis • Autoimmune disease • Neuromuscular junction • Thymectomy

KEY POINTS

- Myasthenia gravis (MG) is an autoimmune disorder caused by antibodies directed at proteins concentrated at the neuromuscular junction, most commonly the acetylcholine receptor.
- MG presents in a highly variable fashion with fluctuating weakness, which ranges in severity from isolated ptosis to life-threatening respiratory collapse.
- MG may be acutely worsened by many commonly used medications, in particular antibiotics, which interfere with neuromuscular transmission.

INTRODUCTION

Myasthenia gravis (MG) is an autoimmune disorder produced by antibodies directed toward postsynaptic proteins concentrated at the neuromuscular junction (NMJ), leading to impaired neuromuscular transmission and consequent fatigable weakness. This characteristic fatigable weakness varies to such an extent that patients may have normal strength during many parts of the day, including during the time of physician examination. Weakness also varies over time with spontaneous remission occurring. This clinical variability and MG's rarity often leads to diagnostic and treatment delay with expected patient frustration. Understanding of MG's pathogenesis has improved over the last few decades and, with that, an appreciation that subtypes of MG based on age, antibody status, and pathologic thymic conditions exist, which allow tailoring of treatment to specific patients. This article discusses the history of MG, its clinical presentation, diagnosis, and clinical classifications. The immunopathogenesis of MG is briefly mentioned and discussed elsewhere. (See Puspa Thapa and Donna L. Farber's article, "The Role of the Thymus in the Immune Response," in this issue.)

HISTORICAL PERSPECTIVE

In 1895, Friedrich Jolly coined the term myasthenia gravis, which was derived from the blending of the Greek *myasthenia*, describing muscle and weakness forming, with the Latin *gravis* for severe.[1,2] The turn of the century brought evidence of an association with thymic hyperplasia and thymoma,

Disclosure Statement: Dr. Kaminski is supported by Muscular Dystrophy Association grant (508240).
Department of Neurology, George Washington University, 2150 Pennsylvania Avenue, NW 9th Floor, Washington, DC 20037, USA
* Corresponding author.
E-mail address: hkaminski@mfa.gwu.edu

Thorac Surg Clin 29 (2019) 133–141
https://doi.org/10.1016/j.thorsurg.2018.12.002

which spurred application of thymus removal as a treatment. Mary Walker[3,4] brought the first truly effective treatment with the administration of physostigmine, a cholinesterase inhibitor, which also supported the contention that MG was caused by a defect of neuromuscular transmission. In the 1950s, John Simpson[5] compiled a range of observations from other diseases and the emerging understanding of the immune system to hypothesize that MG was an autoimmune disorder. The hypothesis received strong support in the early 1970s with the detection of acetylcholine receptor (AChR) antibodies in patient sera and induction of an MG-like condition by immunization of rabbits with purified AChR. In 2000, the muscle-specific kinase (MuSK) was found as an additional autoantigen and, more recently, low-density lipoprotein receptor–related protein 4 (LRP4) has also been identified as a potential autoantibody target.

EPIDEMIOLOGY AND PATIENT CHARACTERISTICS

The incidence of MG is estimated to be 0.04 to 5 with a prevalence of 0.5 to 12.5 per 100,000.[6] A pooling of 55 studies from 1950 to 2007 representing 1.7 billion population-years derived an incidence of 0.53 per 100,000 person-years, and a pooled prevalence of 7.77 cases per 100,000 person-years.[7,8] A European study from 2010 to 2014 suggested that the incidence of MG among individuals older than the age of 60 years was increasing, which was attributed to an increase in elderly population and an overall decreased mortality in the population.[9] Several investigations suggest the incidence of MG is also increasing in the young,[7] as is the case for autoimmune disorders in general. Young MG patients have a higher risk of developing other autoimmune diseases compared with the general population and those with adult-onset MG.[10,11]

MG can occur at any age. Similar to other autoimmune diseases, women are more commonly affected compared with men, with a 2:1 ratio overall. In childbearing years, there is a 3:1 predominance, whereas the ratio is equal before puberty and after age 40 years.[12] Age contributes to defining subgroups of MG. Early-onset MG is variably defined as having an upper age cutoff of 50 years.[13,14] Most patients have serum AChR antibodies with thymic hyperplasia[15] and respond to thymectomy.[16] Individuals with MG older than the age of 50 years (late-onset MG)[14] tend to have thymic atrophy.

PATHOGENESIS

The unifying effector mechanisms of MG are autoantibodies, which target the NMJ, leading to a reduction of AChR concentrated on the postsynaptic muscle surface.[17] The most common autoantibody binds the AChR and is present in about 80% of patients, whereas MuSK antibodies are detected in about 5% and LRP4 in far fewer. This leaves a few patients with no detectable autoantibodies by conventional assays.[17] Such seronegative MG patients may have low levels of antibodies that are not detectable by the current assays or antibodies that bind other components of the NMJ.[1]

Regardless of autoantibody status, the reduction of the AChR coupled with repetitive stimulation or repeated activity leads to inadequate activation of the postsynaptic endplate potential to generate a muscle action potential and thereby the muscle fiber does not contract and weakness occurs. The fatigue observed in patients and the decremental response observed with repetitive stimulation in the electrophysiology laboratory stems from a relative reduction of acetylcholine release, which at normal junctions is not of concern because there is significant reserve to allow an endplate potential to be attained to generate an action potential. In the damaged junction, this reserve is severely compromised.

The autoantibodies of MG compromise AChR concentration by different pathways. AChR antibodies injure the NMJ by 3 mechanisms.[1,18] Antibodies bind to the AChR, which activates the complement cascade forming the membrane attack complex, destroying the postsynaptic membrane. AChR antibodies may crosslink the tightly packed AChR, which leads to their endocytosis and degradation. The muscle cannot compensate with enhanced synthesis of AChR, leading to a reduction in the total number of AChRs on the postsynaptic membrane. AChR antibodies may also compromise the AChR activation, leading to compromised receptor function.[1] In contrast, MuSK and LRP4 are involved in concentration of AChR to the NMJ and autoantibodies to these proteins inhibit signals that cluster AChR on the postsynaptic surface.

Autoantibody production is a function of B cell activity, which further depends on autoantigen-specific T-cell control.[19,20] AChR autoantibody-producing B cells are found in thymus, circulation, lymph nodes, and bone marrow, whereas MuSK antibodies seem not to be synthesized in the thymus.[21] The production of autoantibodies in MG requires the support of CD4+ T cells, which have T helper (Th) lymphocyte function and support autoimmune reaction to autoantigens and activate B cells by secretion of proinflammatory cytokines.[22] In MG patients, several abnormalities of T-cell subsets are appreciated. There is a higher frequency of AChR-specific Th1 and Th17 cells with increased production of interferon-γ and interleukin-17 among MG patients.[23] Thymic and peripheral regulatory T (Treg) cells are also reduced.[24,25] The ratio of follicular Th cells and follicular Treg cells is higher in MG patients, which is consistent with a failure of immune tolerance, which must occur for MG to develop.[26] The persistence of autoreactive lymphocytes seems to critically depend on the expression and antiapoptotic factors, which also support continued survival of cancer cells.

CLINICAL PRESENTATION

The clinical hallmark of MG is the reduction of muscle strength with repetitive activity over minutes to hours; however, the underlying disease severity, hormonal fluctuations, treatments, infections, and unknown factors also produce variations in weakness over weeks to months. Rarely, spontaneous remissions may occur. The disease course is highly variable in patients, especially the initial presentation.[12] After effective therapy is found, patients often realize that symptoms had been present for longer than they originally thought.

Ptosis, diplopia, or both are presenting symptoms in half of MG patients. Ptosis will fluctuate in severity throughout the day and can be unilateral or bilateral. Varying degrees of diplopia or blurred vision occur, which may be vertical, horizontal, or diagonal. Ocular myasthenia is a specific clinical subtype of MG. Upwards of 20% of patient who present with only ocular manifestations will remain with weakness limited to these muscles.[27–29] On examination any combination of extraocular muscle weakness may be appreciated[6] with or without ptosis.[6] A particularly useful examination finding is identification of worsened unilateral ptosis on passive elevation of the contralateral ptotic eyelid.[6] Another characteristic finding, Cogan sign, is present when the eyelid transiently elevates after looking upward from a downward gaze.[6] Almost all patients also have bilateral orbicularis oculi muscle weakness and may have a peek sign manifested by partial opening of the palpebral fissure.[6]

Nearly 80% of patients will have generalized weakness beyond the ocular muscles with variable severity and pattern of muscle involvement. A distinct subgroup of patients has weakness predominantly involving the bulbar muscles producing dysphagia and dysarthria. Facial muscle weakness occurs, which compromises emotional expression and is a source of patient distress. Of particular concern is neck extension weakness, which may be severe enough to compromise breathing and swallowing.[30] Typically, proximal arm muscles are involved more than the legs. Some patients may have highly localized weakness of neck, respiratory, or limb muscles, with no or limited weakness of other muscle groups.[31] Myasthenic crisis is defined as MG-related respiratory muscle weakness so severe that intubation and mechanical ventilation is required.

There are clinical differences between patients with MuSK and AChR antibodies. The peak onset is in the late 30s; however, unlike AChR-MG, it rarely presents in patients older than 70 years.[32] MuSK patients usually present with greater bulbar manifestations and have less pronounced diurnal variations in strength. Atrophy of facial and bulbar muscles with longstanding disease may occur. They also tend to be less responsive to acetylcholinesterase (AChE) inhibitors.[12,33]

DIAGNOSIS
Serum Antibody Testing

The most critical diagnostic test for MG is the serum antibody. AChR antibodies are identified in upwards of 85% of patients with generalized MG and approximately half of patients with purely ocular myasthenia.[7] Three types of assays are commercially available. AChR-binding antibodies are detected using a radioimmunoassay and are the most specific for MG. AChR-blocking and AChR-modulating antibody assays are also available but have no additional diagnostic usefulness and have potential for false-positive results. MuSK antibodies are present in 5% to 8% of MG patients.[17,33] MuSK forms a tetrameric complex with LRP4 on the postsynaptic membrane, and the antibody disrupts AChR clustering dispersion.[32] Antibodies toward LRP4 have been identified in patients with MG with wide variations in prevalence from 3% to almost 20%.[7,9,34] Studies thus far suggest that LRP4-positive patients present younger than age 50 years and are more commonly women compared with non-LRP4 patients.[34] These patients also tend to have milder disease, including presenting with only ocular manifestations. LRP4 antibodies have been identified in patients with multiple sclerosis,[34] neuromyelitis optica,[9,34] and polymyositis,[34] and in upwards of a quarter of amyotrophic lateral sclerosis–affected patients.[34]

There are a few patients who do not have circulating autoantigens. In all likelihood, some of these patients have AChR antibodies that are not detectable by conventional assays but may be confirmed by a cell-based assay, which uses cells that express the AChR in its native form.[17] Other autoantigens may exist, including antibodies to agrin, which is an AChR clustering signal,[7] as well as ColQ protein and cortactin. However, rigorous confirmation has not been performed showing that antibodies to these proteins are pathogenic, which is also true for LRP4.

ELECTRODIAGNOSTICS

Nerve conduction studies with needle electromyography (EMG) are key diagnostic tests of the peripheral nervous system. They are of value to confirm the neurologic examination and exclude other peripheral nervous system disorders. Repetitive electrical stimulation is applied to a peripheral nerve and assessment is made for a reduction in the compound muscle action potential, which confirms the presence of a neuromuscular transmission disorder. In a normal individual, repetitive stimulation has no effect on compound muscle action potential because the amount of acetylcholine is always adequate to trigger the potential. In MG the response becomes decremental with repeated stimulation because the acetylcholine storage becomes depleted.[35] Despite the clear correlation to pathophysiology, the sensitivity of repetitive nerve stimulation in diagnosis of MG is at best 80%.

Other neuromuscular transmission disorders include Lambert-Eaton myasthenic syndrome (LEMS) and botulism. In LEMS, there is an inability to generate the necessary calcium for acetylcholine release owing to the presynaptic voltage-gated calcium channel antibodies and, therefore, there is less amount of acetylcholine released.[35] Hence, an action potential will not be able to be generated when applying low rates of stimulation but high rates of stimulation will increase the compound muscle action potential, leading to an incremental response.[35] Similarly, botulism infection leads to toxin production, which compromises acetylcholine release and shows an incremental response to repetitive stimulation.

The most sensitive electrophysiological approach to confirm a neuromuscular transmission disorder is single-fiber EMG. A sensitivity greater than 90% is reported; however, a systematic review the sensitivity was found to be as low as 66%.[36] Drawbacks of single-fiber EMG is the requirement for an experienced physician and patient cooperation. Single-fiber EMG is highly specific for a neuromuscular transmission disorder, which is most likely to be MG given a clinically consistent presentation. Among patients with other pathologic nerve conditions, a false-positive result may occur.

Clinical Tests

The classic test of intravenous infusion of cholinesterase with unequivocal improvement in weakness, usually of the ocular muscle, is highly specific. Despite the excellent safety record of the edrophonium test, its use has fallen out of favor because of safety concerns. Rarely, severe adverse effects of bradycardia, syncope, and bronchospasm may occur. Gastric upset, excessive lacrimation, and salivation usually happen. Episodic lack of availability of edrophonium in the United States has also become a problem. Estimates of sensitivity vary from is 80% to 95% in ocular MG, which are likely lower in general practice. False positives occur.[37]

Additional tests include the ice pack and rest test. The ice pack test involves applying an ice pack on the patient's drooped eyelid for 5 minutes. The test is positive if there is clinical improvement.[38] For the rest test, patients close their eyes for 20 minutes and are observed for improvement in lid position before and after. Small studies suggest a sensitivity of greater than 90% for these tests but caution needs to be increased in common clinical practice for evaluator and patient bias.

TREATMENT

The following sections discuss the most commonly used therapies for MG (**Table 1**). Treatment guidelines have been established by international consensus and guidelines of neurologic societies of various countries.[39,40] More in-depth discussions have been published.[16,41–65]

Acetylcholinesterase Inhibitors

AChE inhibitors, primarily pyridostigmine bromide, prevent the breakdown of acetylcholine, allowing greater activation of AChR at the damaged NMJ. Pyridostigmine is typically the initial treatment[43] and rarely may suffice as the only treatment of mild weakness.[43] The gastrointestinal adverse effects of nausea, bloating, and diarrhea limit the use of AChE inhibitors. Of particular concern for the intubated patient or those with pulmonary disease are excess respiratory secretions, which may actually worsen breathing.

Thymectomy

Thymus removal has been demonstrated as an effective therapy for patients with generalized, AChR-positive MG who are meet the study criteria of ages of 18 to 65 years.[16] There is insufficient evidence to determine whether MuSK antibody and seronegative patients benefit from

Table 1
Medications and doses used for treatment of myasthenia gravis

Medication	Dosage
Pyridostigmine bromide	30–60 mg q 3–8 h
Extended release pyridostigmine	180 mg qhs
Prednisone	Start with 20 mg/d, increase 5 mg q 3 days, target of 60–80 mg/d
Azathioprine	Start with 50 mg/d, increase 50 mg q 2-4 wk, goal of 1–3 mg/kg/d
Mycophenolate mofetil	1 g twice a day (may increase to 1.5 g twice a day if no improvement in 9 mo)
Tacrolimus	0.035 mg/kg twice a day (trough target 6–9 ng/mL)
Cyclosporin	5 mg/kg/d divided twice a day
Cyclophosphamide	500 mg/m² body surface intravenous monthly
Rituximab	375 mg/m² body surface intravenous weekly for 4 wk, repeated after 6 mo. Pretreat with acetaminophen, diphenhydramine, corticosteroids
Eculizumab	900 mg intravenous weekly for 4 wk, increase to 1200 mg in 5th wk, then 1200 mg q 2 weeks afterward
Plasma exchange	Acute management: remove 1–2 plasma volumes 3 times per week, maximum 6 exchanges
Intravenous immunoglobulin	Acute management: 400 mg/kg/d for 5 d or 1 g/kg/d for 2 d. Pretreat with acetaminophen, diphenhydramine, and normal saline

thymectomy; however, the procedure is not commonly performed on this population.[44] All patients with a thymoma should have the tumor removed unless there are overwhelming medical reasons not to do so.

Corticosteroids

Corticosteroids are the most consistently effective treatment of MG but must be given at high doses for months and then, usually, low doses are taken, often for years.[45] Their use is compromised by their numerous adverse effects. Upwards of 30% of patients respond poorly or are intolerant.[46] The optimal dosing regimen is not known and likely varies by individual, as evidenced by genetic variations affecting treatment response.[47] International consensus guidelines provide options of starting with a high dose (60 mg) or a low dose (10 mg), which is then escalated. Both regimens are followed by a slow taper over many months.[39] An unknown percentage of patients worsen with initiation of prednisone, in particular at high doses; therefore, outpatient regimens typically start at a low dose.

Immunosuppressives

Because of the adverse effects of prednisone, a range of immunosuppressants are used for their steroid-sparing effects. Azathioprine was the first immunosuppressive used. A randomized trial found that corticosteroid dose was reduced after 18 months of treatment compared with placebo.[48] Azathioprine carries the potential for significant hepatotoxicity, myelosuppression, and increased risk of lymphoma with chronic use.[49] Mycophenolate mofetil is also commonly used and is well-tolerated, although severe leukopenia may occur and progressive multifocal leukoencephalopathy is reported with its use.[50] Most importantly, mycophenolate has teratogenic potential, compromising its use in women of childbearing age,[51] and it may increase the risk of malignancy.[52] Since the 1980s, cyclosporine has been used alone or as a steroid-sparing drug[53] but is compromised by significant renal toxicity and hypertension.[53] Tacrolimus has a similar biological mechanism of action but is a superior agent with milder nephrotoxic profile,[54] with 1 retrospective study demonstrating remission for a large percentage patients.[55] Methotrexate is a relatively inexpensive immunosuppressive and a comparison with azathioprine found both drugs to have similar steroid-sparing effects.[56] Hepatotoxicity, anemia, and reversible hair loss may occur with methotrexate.

Acute Therapies

Intravenous immunoglobulin (IVIG) is used in exacerbations of weakness, preoperative preparation, and as a chronic therapy.[57,58] Improvement with

IVIG may be seen within days but controlled studies indicate 3 weeks. IVIG is usually well-tolerated but debilitating headache may occur with and after infusion. Some patients have flu-like symptoms. Urticarial and petechial rash may occur in the days after infusion and many take several weeks to resolve. The greatest concerns are deep venous thrombosis, pulmonary emboli, stroke, or myocardial infarction.[59] There are no known risk factors for their development.

Plasma exchange is performed for the same indications as IVIG[60] and typically involves exchange of 1.5 to 2 blood volumes during a single session performed 3 to 6 times. Benefits of exchange resolve after 6 weeks, if chronic therapy is not instituted. Benefit may be seen within hours but typically over days. In rare patients, plasma exchange may be used as a chronic therapy. Adverse effects include hypotension, nausea, and vomiting due to fluid shifts and electrolyte changes during plasma exchange. The most significant limitations are infections and thrombotic complications caused by the intravenous catheters required for therapy; however, these adverse effects may be reduced by use of peripheral catheters when possible.[60] IVIG therapy may have fewer complications and similar efficacy to plasma exchange.[61]

Complement Inhibition

AChR antibodies injure the NMJ by local activation of complement, which has made for an ideal therapeutic target. Eculizumab is a monoclonal antibody directed against the C5 component of complement and administered by periodic intravenous infusion. In 2017, the US Food and Drug Administration approved its use for AChR antibody–positive, generalized MG. It is not expected that eculizumab would be efficacious for patients without AChR antibodies. Complement inhibition places patients at risk for meningococcal infections and patients require appropriate vaccination before treatment.[62] Eculizumab costs several hundred thousand dollars per year for patients in the United States. Many other countries have not approved its use.

Rituximab

Rituximab is a monoclonal antibody that targets CD20 present on a large number of B cells leading to their elimination.[63] In MuSK antibody-positive patients, rituximab was shown in prospective, controlled trials to reduces prednisone dose, decrease use of immunosuppressants, improve strength, and drop MuSK antibody concentration.[64,65] Case series also suggest efficacy in

AChR antibody MG; however a recent phase 2 study did not show a signal of efficacy. Although rituximab depletes CD20-positive B cells, it does not eliminate plasmablasts or plasma cells that are generating autoantibodies.

PERIOPERATIVE PREPARATION

Optimal care of the patient involves coordinated care by the surgeon, anesthesiologists, critical specialists, and neurologist. Ideally, the patient should be symptom-free before surgery but this may be difficult to achieve, especially for the newly diagnosed MG patient preparing for thymectomy. Preoperative evaluation should include pulmonary function testing and, when needed, formal pulmonary consultation. MG patients are typically on cholinesterase inhibitors for symptomatic relief but their use in the perioperative period may complicate the patient's respiratory status. In particular, the combination with neuromuscular blocking agents may put the patient at high risk for developing postoperative respiratory complications.[66] Corticosteroids may be required to optimize strength but may compromise wound healing. To optimize strength immediately before surgery, plasma exchange or IVIG is often used.

Table 2
Drugs to use with caution

Category of Medications	Medications Associated with Clinical Worsening of MG
Antiarrhythmic	Procainamide, quinidine, verapamil, propafenone
Antibiotic	Aminoglycosides, fluoroquinolones, azithromycin, clindamycin, telithromycin
Antiepileptic	Carbamazepine, gabapentin, phenytoin
Antimalarial	Chloroquine, quinine
Beta blockers	Propranolol, timolol
Checkpoint inhibitors	Pembrolizumab, nivolumab, ipilimumab
Neuropsychiatric	Lithium, trimethadione
Miscellaneous	Botulinum toxin, D-penicillamine, interferon-alpha, magnesium, oral contraceptive pills

There are no data supporting which may be superior.[66] The choice between IVIG versus plasma exchange depends on the patient's history, taking into account if there are any contraindications to treatment, hospital resources, or patient preference. Although limiting postoperative complications is best performed by optimization of clinical status before operation, the care team should be vigilant regarding respiratory decompensation that may occur even with excellent preoperative care.

Neuromuscular transmission is compromised by many medications (**Table 2**) and, in the MG patient, exposure to certain drugs may induce rapid, life-threatening weakness.[67] In addition to drugs that affect neuromuscular transmission, there are agents that induce an autoimmune response. The most important and recently identified are the class of cancer treatments designed to bypass the immune systems checkpoints to eliminate neoplasms.[68] Patients have been found to develop de novo MG or produce severe exacerbations with known MG.[68]

SUMMARY

MG is a difficult disease to identify clinically; however, when recognized, simple serum autoantibody testing will confirm diagnosis in most patients. Additional evaluation by an experienced neurologist using electrophysiological testing will confirm diagnosis in the remaining patients. A wide range of treatment options exist, which usually includes thymectomy, corticosteroids, and immunosuppression; however, these need to be tailored to patient subgroups. The patient with MG has special needs, in particular awareness of medications that may significantly exacerbate weakness, as well as systemic infections. This is particularly important in the perioperative period when additional acute therapies of IVIG and plasma exchange may be used to optimize strength. MG remains a grave disease. Therapies have improved care but patients are compromised by significant adverse effects.

REFERENCES

1. Katirji B, Kaminski HJ, Ruff RL, editors. Neuromuscular disorders in clinical practice. New York: Springer Science & Business Media; 2013.
2. Keesey J. Myasthenia gravis. An illustrated history. Roseville (CA): Publisher's Design Group; 2002.
3. Walker MB. Treatment of myasthenia gravis with physostigmine. Lancet 1934;1(5779):1200–1.
4. Walker MB. Case showing the effect of prostigmin on myasthenia gravis. Proc R Soc Med 1935;28: 759–61.
5. Simpson JA. Myasthenia gravis, a new hypothesis. Scot Med J 1960;5:419–36.
6. Smith SV, Lee AG. Update on ocular myasthenia gravis. Neurol Clin 2017;35:115–23.
7. Binks S, Vincent A, Palace J. Myasthenia gravis: a clinical-immunological update. J Neurol 2016;263: 826–34.
8. Carr AS, Cardwell CR, McCarron PO, et al. A systemic review of population based epidemiological studies in myasthenia gravis. BMC Neurol 2010; 18:46.
9. Zieda A, Ravina K, Giazere I, et al. A nationwide epidemiological study of myasthenia gravis in Latvia. Eur J Neurol 2018;25:519–26.
10. Popperud TH, Boldingh MI, Rasmussen M, et al. Juvenile myasthenia gravis in Norway: clinical characteristics, treatment, and long-term outcome in a nation-wide population-based cohort 2017;21: 707–18.
11. Huang X, Li Y, Feng H, et al. Clinical characteristics of juvenile myasthenia gravis in Southern China. Front Neurol 2018;9(77):1–7.
12. Kuks, Jan BM. Clinical presentation and epidemiology of myasthenia gravis. In: Kaminski HJ, Kusner LL, editors. Myasthenia gravis and related disorders. 3rd edition. New York: Humana Press; 2018. p. 85–100.
13. Pakzad Z, Aziz T, Oger J. Increasing incidence of myasthenia gravis among elderly in British Columbia, Canada. Neurology 2011;76(17):1526–8.
14. Evoli A, Batocchi AP, Minisci C, et al. Clinical characteristics and prognosis of myasthenia gravis in older people. J Am Geriatr Soc 2000;48(11):1442–8.
15. Marx A, Pfister F, Schalke B, et al. The different roles of thymus in the pathogenesis of the various myasthenia gravis subtypes. Autoimmun Rev 2013;12: 875–84.
16. Wolfe GI, Kaminski HJ, Aban IB, et al. Randomized trial of thymectomy in myasthenia gravis. N Engl J Med 2016;375:511–22.
17. Le Panse R, Berrih-Aknin S. Immunopathogenesis of Myasthenia Gravis. In: Kaminski HJ, Kusner LL, editors. Myasthenia gravis and related disorders. 3rd edition. New York: Humana Press; 2018. p. 47–60.
18. Kusner LL, Kaminski HJ, Soltys J. Effect of complement and its regulation on myasthenia gravis pathogenesis. Expert Rev Clin Immunol 2008;4:43–52.
19. Le Panse R, Berrih-Aknin S. Autoimmune myasthenia gravis: autoantibody mechanisms and new developments on immune regulation. Curr Opin Neurol 2013;26:569–76.
20. Yi JS, Guptill JT, Stathopoulos P, et al. B cells in the pathophysiology of myasthenia gravis. Muscle Nerve 2018;57:172–84.
21. Leite MI, Strobel P, Jones M, et al. Fewer thymic changes in MuSK antibody-positive than in MuSK antibody-negative MG. Ann Neurol 2005;57:444–8.

22. Fan X, Lin C, Han J, et al. Follicular helper CD4+ T cells in human neuroautoimmune diseases and their animal models. Mediators Inflamm 2015;2015: 638968.

23. Cao Y, Amezquita RA, Kleinstein SH, et al. Autoreactive T cells from patients with Myasthenia Gravis are characterized by elevated IL-17, IFN-gamma, and GM-CSF and diminished IL-10 production. J Immunol 2016;196:2075–84.

24. Alahgholi-Hajibehzad M, Kasapoglu P, Jafari R, et al. The role of T regulatory cells in immunopathogenesis of myasthenia gravis: implications for therapeutics. Expert Rev Clin Immunol 2015;11:859–70.

25. Alahgholi-Hajibehzad M, Oflazer P, Aysal F, et al. Regulatory function of CD4+CD25++ T cells in patients with myasthenia gravis is associated with phenotypic changes and STAT5 signaling: 1,25-Dihydroxyvitamin D3 modulates the suppressor activity. J Neuroimmunol 2015;281:51–60.

26. Wen Y, Yang B, Lu J, et al. Imbalance of circulating CD4(+)CXCR5(+)FOXP3(+) Tfr-like cells and CD4(+)CXCR5(+)FOXP3(-) Tfh-like cells in myasthenia gravis. Neurosci Lett 2016;630:176–82.

27. Gilhus NE. Myasthenia gravis. N Engl J Med 2017; 376(13):e25.

28. Grob D, Brunner N, Namba T, et al. Lifetime course of myasthenia gravis. Muscle Nerve 2008;37:141–9.

29. Mazzoli M, Ariatti A, Valzania F, et al. Factors affecting outcome in ocular myasthenia gravis. Int J Neurosci 2018;128:15–24.

30. Romano AE, Al-Qudah Z, Kaminski HJ, et al. Concurrent paraspinous myopathy and myasthenia gravis. J Clin Neuromuscul Dis 2017;18:218–22.

31. Alshekhlee A, Miles JD, Katirji B, et al. Incidence and mortality rates of myasthenia gravis and myasthenic crisis in US hospitals. Neurology 2009;72: 1548–54.

32. Evoli A, Alboini PE, Iorio R. Pattern of ocular involvement in myasthenia gravis with MuSK antibodies. J Neurol Neurosurg Psychiatry 2017;88:761–3.

33. Evoli A, Alboini PE, Damato V, et al. Myasthenia gravis with antibodies to MuSK: an update. Ann N Y Acad Sci 2018;1412:82–9.

34. Bacchi S, Kramer P, Chalk C. Autoantibodies to low-density lipoprotein receptor-related double seronegative myasthenia gravis: a systemic review. Can J Neurol Sci 2018;45:62–7.

35. Preston DC, Shapiro BE. Repetitive nerve stimulation. In: Preston DC, Shapiro BE, editors. Electromyography and neuromuscular disorders. 3rd edition. New York: Elsevier Health; 2013. p. 52–61.

36. Kouyoumdjian JA, Stalberg E. Stimulated jitter with concentric needle in 42 myasthenia gravis patients. Arq Neuropsiquiatr 2013;71:237–43.

37. Evoli A, Tonali P, Bartoccioni AP, et al. Ocular myasthenia: diagnostic and therapeutic problems. Acta Neurol Scand 1988;77:31–5.

38. Fakiri MO, Tavy DL, Hama-Amin AD, et al. Accuracy of the ice test in the diagnosis of myasthenia gravis in patients with ptosis. Muscle Nerve 2013;48:902–4.

39. Sanders DB, Wolfe GI, Benatar M, et al. International consensus guidance for management of myasthenia gravis: executive summary. Neurology 2016;87: 419–25.

40. Sussman J, Farrugia MF, Maddison P, et al. Myasthenia gravis: association of British neurologists' management guidelines. Pract Neurol 2015;15: 199–206.

41. Kaminski HJ. Treatment of myasthenia gravis. In: Kaminski HJ, Kusner LL, editors. Myasthenia gravis and related disorders. 3rd edition. New York: Humana Press; 2018. p. 169–87.

42. Farmakidis C, Pasnoor M, Dimachkie MM, et al. Treatment of myasthenia gravis. Neurol Clin 2018; 36:311–37.

43. Maggi L, Mantegazza R. Treatment of myasthenia gravis: focus on pyridostigmine. Clin Drug Investig 2011;31:691–701.

44. Yuan HK, Huang BS, Kung SY, et al. The effectiveness of thymectomy on seronegative generalized myasthenia gravis: comparing with seropositive cases. Acta Neurol Scand 2007;115:181–4.

45. Pascuzzi RM, Coslett HB, Johns TR. Long-term corticosteroid treatment of myasthenia gravis: report of 116 patients. Ann Neurol 1984;15:291–8.

46. Cosi V, Citterio A, Lombardi M, et al. Effectiveness of steroid treatment in myasthenia gravis: a retrospective study. Acta Neurol Scand 1991;84:33–9.

47. Xie Y, Li HF, Sun L, et al. The role of osteopontin and its gene on glucocorticoid response in myasthenia gravis. Front Neurol 2017;8:1–9.

48. Palace J, Newsome-Davis J. A randomized double blind trial of prednisolone alone or with azathioprine in myasthenia gravis. Neurology 1998;50:1778–83.

49. Pedersen EG, Pottegard A, Hallas J, et al. Use of azathioprine for nonthymoma myasthenia and risk of cancer: a nationwide case-control study in Denmark. Eur J Neurol 2013;20:942–8.

50. Termsarasab P, Katirji B. Opportunistic infections in myasthenia gravis treated with mycophenolate mofetil. J Neuroimmunol 2012;249:83–5.

51. Coscia LA, Armenti DP, King RW, et al. Update on the teratogenicity of maternal mycophenolate mofetil. J Pediatr Genet 2015;4:42–55.

52. Vernino S, Salomao DR, Habermann TM, et al. Primary CNS lymphoma complicating treatment of myasthenia gravis with mycophenolate mofetil. Neurology 2005;65:639–41.

53. Ciafaloni E, Nikhar NK, Massey JM, et al. Retrospective analysis of the use of cyclosporine in myasthenia gravis. Ann N Y Acad Sci 1993;681:539–51.

54. Cruz JL, Wolff ML, Vanderman AJ. The emerging role of tacrolimus in myasthenia gravis. Therap Adv Neurol Dis 2015;8:92–103.

55. Tao X, Wang W, Jing F, et al. Long-term efficacy and side effects of low-dose tacrolimus for the treatment of myasthenia gravis. Neurol Sci 2017;38:325–30.

56. Heckmann JM, Rawoot A, Bateman K, et al. A single-blinded trial of methotrexate versus azathioprine as steroid-sparing agents in generalized myasthenia gravis. BMC Neurol 2011;11:97.

57. Zinman L, Ng E, Bril V. IV immunoglobulin in patients with myasthenia gravis: a randomized controlled trial. Neurology 2007;68:837–41.

58. Elenbroker C, Seitz F, Spengler A, et al. Intravenous immunoglobulin maintenance treatment in myasthenia gravis: a randomized, controlled trial sample size simulation. Muscle Nerve 2014;50:999–1004.

59. Paran D, Herishanu Y, Elkayam O, et al. Venous and arterial thrombosis following administration of intravenous immunoglobulins. Blood Coagul Fibrinolysis 2005;16:313–8.

60. Guptill JT, Oakley D, Kuchibhatla M, et al. A retrospective study of complications of therapeutic plasma exchange in myasthenia. Muscle Nerve 2013;47:170–6.

61. Ferrero B, Durelli L. High-dose intravenous immunoglobulin G treatment of myasthenia gravis. Neurol Sci 2002;1:S9–24.

62. Howard JF Jr, Utsugisawa K, Benatar M, et al. Safety and efficacy of eculizumab in anti-acetylcholine receptor antibody-positive refractory generalised myasthenia gravis (REGAIN): a phase 3, randomised, double-blind, placebo-controlled, multicentre study. Lancet Neurol 2017;16:976–86.

63. Chambers SA, Isenberg D. Anti-B cell therapy (rituximab) in the treatment of autoimmune diseases. Lupus 2005;14:210–4.

64. Diaz-Manera J, Martinez-Hernandez E, Querol L, et al. Long-lasting treatment effect of rituximab in MuSK myasthenia. Neurology 2012;78:189–93.

65. Hehir MK, Hobson-Webb LD, Benatar M, et al. Rituximab as treatment for anti-MuSK myasthenia gravis: multicenter blinded prospective review. Neurology 2017;89:1069–77.

66. Sonett J, Bromberger B, Jaretzki A III. Thymectomy for non-thymomatous myasthenia gravis. In: Kaminski HJ, Kusner LL, editors. Myasthenia gravis and related disorders. 3rd edition. New York: Humana Press; 2018. p. 199–219.

67. Howard JF Jr. Toxic neuromuscular transmission disorders. In: Kaminski HJ, Kusner LL, editors. Myasthenia gravis and related disorders. 3rd edition. New York: Humana Press; 2018. p. 275–98.

68. Algaeed M, Mukharesh L, Heinzelmann M, et al. Pearls and oysters: case report: pembrolizumab induced myasthenia gravis. Neurology 2018;91:1–3.

A Neurologist's Perspective on Thymectomy for Myasthenia Gravis
Current Perspective and Future Trials

Wentao Mi, MD, PhD, Nicholas J. Silvestri, MD,
Gil I. Wolfe, MD*

KEYWORDS

- Myasthenia gravis • Generalized • Acetylcholine receptor antibody • Thymectomy
- Neurology perspective

KEY POINTS

- Transsternal thymectomy confers several benefits in the management of generalized, acetylcholine receptor antibody–positive myasthenia gravis.
- These benefits include improved clinical status, reduced need for corticosteroids and other immunosuppressive agents, reduced side effects from medications, and fewer hospital admissions for management of disease exacerbations.
- It is anticipated that other surgical approaches staged with the intention to remove as much thymic tissue as possible would confer similar benefits.
- The benefits of thymectomy extend for at least 5 years after the procedure.

INTRODUCTION

Myasthenia gravis (MG) is an acquired disorder of neuromuscular transmission manifested by fluctuations in severity of muscle weakness and fatigue. Myasthenic weakness typically affects skeletal muscles, including ocular, bulbar, and proximal extremity muscles. Respiratory muscles are impacted in severe cases. It is an autoimmune disease most commonly caused by autoantibodies against the nicotinic acetylcholine receptors (AChRs). In the past 15 years, additional autoantibodies directed against other proteins localized to the postsynaptic membrane have been implicated in the disease. Inhibition of the hydrolysis of acetylcholine neurotransmitter in the synaptic cleft or moderating the blocking or destruction of AChRs is a primary medical strategy of MG treatment. The main modalities in MG management include symptomatic treatment with anticholinesterase inhibitors (pyridostigmine), immunotherapy with immunosuppressants (corticosteroids, azathioprine, mycophenolate mofetil, cyclosporine, methotrexate, and tacrolimus), immunomodulators (plasmapheresis and intravenous immunoglobulin), monoclonal antibodies (eculizumab and

Disclosure Statement: Dr G.I. Wolfe serves as an advisor and speaker and has received research funding from Alexion Pharmaceuticals. The MGTX thymectomy trial was funded by National Institutes of Health/National Institute of Neurological Disorders and Stroke (U01 NS042685), Muscular Dystrophy Association, and Myasthenia Gravis Foundation of America. Dr N.J. Silvestri has served as an advisor for Alexion Pharmaceuticals. Dr W. Mi has no conflicts of interest.
Department of Neurology, Jacobs School of Medicine and Biomedical Sciences, University at Buffalo/SUNY, 1010 Main Street, 2nd Floor, Buffalo, NY 14202, USA
* Corresponding author.
E-mail address: gilwolfe@buffalo.edu

Thorac Surg Clin 29 (2019) 143–150
https://doi.org/10.1016/j.thorsurg.2018.12.003
1547-4127/19/© 2019 Elsevier Inc. All rights reserved.

rituximab, targeting complement activation cells and B cells, respectively); and surgical treatment with thymectomy.[1]

The benefit of thymectomy in MG was first reported in 1939 by Dr Alfred Blalock and colleagues,[2] who observed marked and sustained improvement for several years after removal of a cystic thymic tumor in a 21-year-old woman. They then proposed exploration of the thymic region in all patients with severe MG.[3] In 1941, Blalock and colleagues[4] performed transsternal thymectomy on 6 nonthymomatous MG patients. One patient became asymptomatic 2 months postoperation, 2 significantly improved, 3 saw mild benefit, and 1 died of respiratory failure 3 days after surgery.[4] Subsequently, Blalock's team operated on 20 MG patients, further solidifying a role for surgery in management of MG.[5] Thymectomy was routinely used for MG by the 1940s. Over the next 70 years, hundreds of clinical observations and studies reported an overall positive outcome of thymectomy in nonthymomatous MG. The actual benefits, however, remained in question and were the source of skepticism, and there were repeated calls for formal prospective studies.[6–8]

In 2000, Gronseth and Barohn[9] performed a comprehensive systemic review of 310 publications on MG and thymectomy and identified 21 class II MG cohorts reporting outcomes in patients treated with or without thymectomy. Most studies demonstrated a favorable response from thymectomy in rates of remission and improvement. The outcomes were mainly based on retrospective and uncontrolled studies and, therefore, entertained risks of bias. Methodologic flaws in study design created concern in drawing conclusions. These flaws included varying definitions for remission, different surgical approaches with some not well described, poor matching of subjects to surgical and medication-only arms, and no standardized medical therapies. The review concluded that thymectomy should be considered a treatment option in nonthymomatous MG and joined the chorus of investigators calling for a randomized controlled trial.

To address the thymectomy dilemma, the randomized Thymectomy Trial in Non-Thymomatous Myasthenia Gravis Patients Receiving Prednisone Therapy (MGTX) was designed to answer 3 questions: (1) Is thymectomy plus prednisone superior to prednisone alone regarding symptomatic improvement? (2) Can thymectomy lower the total therapeutic dose of prednisone? and (3) Will thymectomy, by lowering prednisone or other immunosuppressive agent requirements, result in a lower side-effect burden for patients?[10,11]

DESIGN OF THYMECTOMY TRIAL IN NON-THYMOMATOUS MYASTHENIA GRAVIS PATIENTS RECEIVING PREDNISONE THERAPY

The MGTX study was an international, single (rater)-blinded, randomized trial to compare the outcome of extended transsternal thymectomy plus prednisone (surgical arm) versus the identical prednisone protocol alone (nonsurgical arm) in generalized nonthymomatous MG. Patients were recruited from 67 centers in 18 countries on 6 continents between 2006 and 2012. Inclusion criteria included women and men between ages 18 years and 65 years diagnosed within the past 5 years, Myasthenia Gravis Foundation of America (MGFA) clinical classification II through IV at entry, AChR antibody–positive, and receiving appropriate anticholinesterase treatment with or without oral prednisone. Approximately 7000 patients were screened across the centers. Sites were asked to consider every MG patient they encountered. A total of 126 patients were randomized, with 66 in the surgical and 60 in the nonsurgical arms.

This study was designed to overcome methodological flaws identified in analysis of prior series.[9] First, patients were randomized so that patients in both treatment groups would have similar baseline demographic and clinical characteristics. Second, outcome rating was performed in a blinded fashion—subjects were repeatedly instructed not to disclose whether or not they had surgery to these evaluators and wore high-collared jerseys that were provided by the study. Third, a standardized prednisone dosing protocol was used, with fixed increases or decreases in dosing based on whether a subject had achieved and maintained the MGFA definition of minimal manifestation status (MMS).[12] This ensured that subjects in both arms would be subjected to as identical a medication regimen as possible. Fourth, a dual primary outcome measure developed in concert with National Instiute of Neurological Disorders and Stroke/National Institutes of Health included time-weighted average quantitative myasthenia gravis (QMG) scores and time-weighted average required prednisone doses over a 3-year period. This 2-staged evaluation ensured that incorrect conclusions about the impact of thymectomy would be avoided. For instance, if the thymectomy group had better clinical status outcomes on the time-weighted QMG but at the cost of higher prednisone exposure, the dual primary outcome approach would temper enthusiasm for the surgery.

Prednisone was administered on alternate days (ADs) in all subjects. Because patients entered with symptomatic disease based on MGFA clinical classifications, prednisone was increased by 10 mg on ADs until MMS was achieved, with a peak dose of 100 mg, ADs, escalating to 120 mg, ADs, if MMS was still not present at month 4. In addition to the requirement of MMS, the QMG score had to be less than14 and at least 1 point below baseline prior to tapering. Tapering was by 10 mg every 2 weeks until a dose of 40 mg, ADs, was reached and then slowed to 5 mg every month as long as MMS was maintained.[11]

THYMECTOMY APPROACH

The purpose of thymectomy in MG is to remove as completely as possible the thymus gland. This objective is challenged by the complicated anatomy of the thymus, which consists of noncontiguous, multilobular tissue interspersed with fat in the neck and mediastinum. Four surgical approaches are commonly used: transsternal, transcervical, minimally invasive video-assisted with or without robotic assistance, and a combined transcervical-transsternal approach.[13] For MGTX, an extended transsternal approach was chosen, given its familiarity to surgeons across centers and the goal of ensuring an en bloc resection of all mediastinal tissue that could anatomically contain gross and/or microscopic thymus.[14] Careful consideration before and during the trial was made to allow for the growing practice of minimally invasive thymectomy approaches but ultimately rejected in light of the concern that a negative result for the surgical arm with such allowance would raise serious questions on whether an adequate thymic resection was actually performed.

CLINICAL OUTCOME

The outcome of the trial was assessed by 2 primary endpoints, the time-weighted average QMG score and prednisone dosing requirements over a period of 3 years. Patients who underwent thymectomy had a lower (more favorable) time-weighted average QMG score than those who received prednisone alone (6.15 ± 4.09 vs 8.99 ± 4.93; 95% CI, 0.47–5.22; $P<.001$ [**Table 1**]). This QMG score difference exceeded a threshold of 2.3 points found indicative of clinical improvement.[15] Furthermore, the thymectomy group's AD prednisone requirements to maintain MMS over the 3 years was also significantly lower than the medication-only arm (32 mg ± 23 mg vs 54 mg ± 29 mg; 95% CI, 12–32; $P<.001$ [see **Table 1**]). In other words, thymectomy not only produced a better clinical outcome but also did so

with lower prednisone requirements. The benefit of thymectomy could be discerned within the first 6 months after randomization, becoming more prominent later in the first year. It is important to realize that both patient groups improved over time based on QMG scores, but the thymectomy group did so more robustly. The beneficial impact of thymectomy persisted through the next 2 years of the main part of the study. Prespecified subgroup analyses demonstrated that the benefits of thymectomy were independent of gender or age above or below 40 years at MG onset, at least for 1 component of the dual primary outcome (see **Table 1**).

Secondary outcome measures provided further support for the benefit of thymectomy in nonthymomatous MG. Patient-reported surveys regarding treatment-associated symptoms showed that the thymectomy group fared better from the standpoint of subjects with symptoms ($P<.001$), total number of symptoms ($P<.001$), and distress level related to symptoms ($P = .003$) over the 3-year period. The thymectomy arm also demonstrated a significant reduction in hospital admissions (9% vs 37%; $P<.001$). No significant difference was seen, however, in a treatment-associated complications survey completed by investigators.

The need for additional immunosuppressive agents—allowed after the first year for patients who had not yet achieved MMS or who were burdened by significant side effects of corticosteroids—was also significantly reduced by thymectomy. Intravenous immunoglobulin delivery to manage disease exacerbations was also significantly lower in the thymectomy group (see **Table 1**). The time-weighted MG activities of daily living (MG-ADL) score also was significantly lower (more favorable) for the thymectomy arm ($P = .008$) as was the percentage of patients achieving MMS at month 12 (67% vs 37%; $P = .001$), month 24 (66% vs 38%; $P = .003$), and month 36 (67% vs 47%; $P = .03$ [see **Table 1**]).

THYMECTOMY APPROACHES AND COMPLICATIONS

Extended transsternal thymectomy proved to be well tolerated in the trial, and thymic resection in general has an excellent track record of safety in MG.[16] In MGTX, postoperative recovery was uneventful in most patients. A surgical complication was seen in only 1 of 66 patients. The extended transsternal thymectomy procedure used in the trial removes all visible mediastinal thymic lobes and most mediastinal perithymic fat, including resection in pericardial vena caval, phrenic,

Table 1
Summary of results from the randomized thymectomy trial in myasthenia gravis

Outcome	Thymectomy Plus Prednisone		Prednisone Alone		Estimated Difference	P Value
	Measure (mean ±SD)	No. of Patients	Measure (mean ±SD)	No. of Patients	(95% CI)[a]	
Primary outcome analyses						
Time-weighted average QMG score over 3-year period (overall)[b]	6.15 ± 4.09	62	8.99 ± 4.93	56	2.85 (0.47–5.22)	<0.001
QMG score by age at MG onset						
<40 y[c]	6.50 ± 4.41	42	9.60 ± 5.32	34	3.10 (−0.13–6.33)	0.007
>40 y[c]	5.33 ± 2.79	18	7.85 ± 3.50	18	2.52 (−0.65–5.69)	0.02
QMG score by gender						
Female[c]	6.47 ± 4.13	46	9.73 ± 5.16	38	3.26 (0.34–6.18)	0.002
Male[c]	5.23 ± 3.95	16	7.45 ± 4.11	18	2.22 (−1.96–6.40)	0.12
Time-weighted average alternative-day prednisone dose over 3-year period (overall)[b]	32 ± 23	61	54 ± 29	56	22 (12–32)	<0.001
Prednisone dose by age at MG onset						
<40 y[c]	35 ± 25	41	55 ± 30	33	20 (8–33)	0.002
>40 y[c]	27 ± 18	18	49 ± 29	19	23 (7–39)	0.007
Prednisone dose by gender						
Female[c]	33 ± 25	45	54 ± 27	37	21 (9–32)	<0.001
Male[c]	31 ± 18	16	55 ± 34	19	24 (5–42)	0.01
Secondary outcome analyses						
Time-weighted average MG-ADL (over 3-year period)[d]	2.24 ± 2.09	61	3.41 ± 2.58	55	1.17 (0.31–2.03)	0.008
MMS (% of patients in MMS)						

At 12 mo[e]	67%	61	37%	54	30.2% (12.7%–47.6%)	0.001
At 24 mo[e]	66%	59	38%	53	28.4% (10.6%–46.2%)	0.003
At 36 mo[e]	67%	58	47%	51	20.2% (1.9%–33.5%)	0.03
Intravenous immunoglobulin use, no. of patients (%)[e]	11 (17%)	65	23 (40%)	58	22.7% (7%–38.3%)	0.005
Azathioprine use, no. of patients (%)[e]	11 (17%)	65	28 (48%)	58	31.4% (15.6%–47.1%)	<0.001
Adverse events						
No. of events[f]	48	66	93	60	NA	<0.001
Hospitalization, no. of patients (%)[g]	15 (23%)	66	31 (52%)	60	NA	<0.01

a A 95% CI was used in all analyses except for analyses involving the QMG score, for which a 99.5% CI was applied.
b P values for between-group comparisons are based on 2 independent sample Student t tests.
c P values for interaction with treatment were based on fitting a general linear model separately for each variable (age at MG onset or gender).
d P value based on 2 sample t test. MG-ADL scores 0, 1, 2, and 3, where 0 = normal and higher scores are worse.
e P values are based on logistic regression.
f The P value is based on Poisson regression that included all 126 patients.
g The P value is based on a chi-square test that included all 126 patients.

diaphragmatic, and cervical areas.[12,13] The world-wide spread of minimally invasive thymectomy techniques is a rational development in light of the accelerated postoperative recovery, reduced blood loss, improved cosmesis, and reduced pain observed in these approaches. MG outcomes from both transcervical and video-assisted thoracoscopic approaches that avoid a median sternotomy have rivaled those seen in more invasive procedures, with similar specimen weights retrieved.[17-19] MGTX was planned and completed during an era of dissemination and refinement of minimally invasive techniques. As discussed previously, it was decided to not introduce these newer approaches in the trial, given concern related to the extent of residual[12] or ectopic thymic tissue.[20] Prior reports argue that incomplete resections are associated with lower remission rates and may require repeat operations.[21-23] A large study has reported the negative impact on MG outcomes of ectopic thymic tissue found in thymectomy specimens resected from nonthymomatous MG patients, again making the case that the resection should be as complete as can be safely performed.[20] Nevertheless, the authors speculate that MG patients should derive a similar constellation of benefits from minimally invasive approaches as long as the surgical team's intent is to perform as complete a thymectomy as possible.[24] Randomized trials testing different techniques represent an ideal situation but are challenging in concept and would take years to perform. Video-assisted thoracoscopic procedures now prevail at many of the MGTX trial sites.

FUTURE PERSPECTIVES ON MYASTHENIA GRAVIS MANAGEMENT

Thymectomy remains a mainstay of treatment in thymomatous MG and nonthymomatous MG, particularly in patients harboring elevated levels of AChR antibodies. A US-based study that utilized the Nationwide Inpatient Sample database documented a declining trend in the rate of MG hospitalizations for an actual thymectomy, with such admissions falling from 7% in 2000 to 1.5% in 2005.[25] The authors suspect the decline was related to health care providers waiting for more definitive evidence from MGTX as well as the expansion of other therapeutic strategies for treating the disease. The same inpatient analysis demonstrated a marked increase of MG admissions for intravenous immunoglobulin.[25]

Although MGTX enrolled the largest subpopulation of MG—that is, generalized patients with elevated AChR antibodies[26]—it is important to point out that there are limitations in generalizing

the trial's conclusions. First, subjects tended to be younger, and post hoc analyses failed to demonstrate a benefit for thymectomy for the few patients who were above age 50 years at enrollment.[11] It is the younger patients with MG who most commonly demonstrate the thymic follicular hyperplasia linked to several lines of evidence pointing to the thymus playing a central role in MG disease generation.[27,28] The thymus undergoes fatty replacement in middle age and beyond, and antigen-specific T cells are barely seen in atrophied thymus.[29] A satellite study that performed detailed histologic analysis on resected thymus specimens from MGTX failed to correlate disease outcomes with the degree of thymic hyperplasia.[30] After investigating a variety of outcomes, the 1 correlation that stood out was a greater time-weighted prednisone requirement in patients with greater intrathymic fat content. MGTX, as a result, does not provide a simple guide to predict outcomes after surgery based on findings from chest imaging or even histologic inspection of the thymus after resection.

Other limitations in extending results from MGTX to the larger MG population include the trial limiting disease duration to no more than 5 years; the mean disease duration was just over 1 year. There is a consensus to perform thymectomy as early as possible in the disease course. MGTX certainly does not challenge this notion. It could be argued that more liberal use of corticosteroid-sparing immunosuppressive agents could have moderated or eliminated the improved clinical outcomes seen with thymectomy. Randomized trials in MG of such agents, however, have failed to demonstrate this type of improvement when the drug was added to prednisone.[31,32]

MGTX did not enroll seronegative patients or those with other antibody subtypes. Numerous series have failed to demonstrate a convincing benefit for thymectomy in MG patients with antibodies to muscle-specific kinase (MuSK) or lipoprotein receptor–related protein 4 (LRP4).[26,33-35] The international consensus guidance for MG management does not recommend thymectomy in patients with MuSK, LRP4, or agrin antibodies.[36] MGTX enrolled subjects above 18 years and cannot directly inform decisions for the juvenile MG population. The international consensus guidance does support the use of thymectomy in this age group if medical treatment response is inadequate or if potential or real complications of immunotherapy are too great.[36] It does provide caution, however, for the need to carefully exclude congenital myasthenic or other neuromuscular syndromes in seronegative juvenile patients prior to proceeding with thymectomy.

Finally, pure ocular MG patients were not enrolled in MGTX. Thymectomy for ocular MG remains an area of controversy, and results from studies and meta-analyses question whether there are actual benefits.[9,37-42]

SUMMARY

MGTX provided answers to questions and allayed doubts about the impact of thymectomy in nonthymomatous MG that have persisted for approximately 75 years. The trial demonstrated that, through 3 years, extended transsternal thymectomy plus prednisone confers benefits over prednisone alone from the standpoint of improved clinical outcomes, reduced requirements for immunosuppressive medications and hospitalizations, and decreased distress reported by patients related to side effects of medication. Several important questions remain unanswered, but MGTX firmly established the important role thymectomy should continue to play in managing the many patients with generalized MG.

REFERENCES

1. Farmakidis C, Pasnoor M, Dimachkie MM, et al. Treatment of myasthenia gravis. Neurol Clin 2018; 36(2):311-37.
2. Blalock A, Mason MF, Morgan HJ, et al. Myasthenia gravis and tumors of the thymic region: report of a case in which the tumor was removed. Ann Surg 1939;110:544-61.
3. Kirschner PA. Alfred Blalock and thymectomy for myasthenia gravis. Ann Thorac Surg 1987;43(3): 348-9.
4. Blalock A, Harvey AM, Ford FR, et al. The treatment of myasthenia gravis by removal of the thymus gland. JAMA 1941;117:1529-33.
5. Blalock A. Thymectomy in the treatment of myasthenia gravis. Report of twenty cases. J Thorac Surg 1944;13:316-39.
6. Oosterhuis HJ. Observations of the natural history of myasthenia gravis and the effect of thymectomy. Ann N Y Acad Sci 1981;377:678-90.
7. Cea G, Benatar M, Verdugo RJ, et al. Thymectomy for non-thymomatous myasthenia gravis (review). Cochrane Libr 2013;10:1-20.
8. Lanska DJ. Indications for thymectomy in myasthenia gravis. Neurology 1990;40:1828-9.
9. Gronseth GS, Barohn RJ. Thymectomy for nonthymomatous autoimmune myasthenia gravis (an evidence-based review). Neurology 2000;55:7-15.
10. Newsom-Davis J, Cutter G, Wolfe GI, et al. Status of the thymectomy trial for nonthymomatous myasthenia gravis patients receiving prednisone. Ann NY Acad Sci 2008;1132:344-7.
11. Wolfe GI, Kaminski HJ, Aban IB, et al. Randomized trial of thymectomy in myasthenia gravis. N Engl J Med 2016;376:511-22.
12. Jaretzki A III, Barohn RJ, Ernstoff RM, et al. Myasthenia gravis: recommendations for clinical research standards. Neurology 2000;55:16-23.
13. Jaretzki A III, Barohn RJ, Engel WK, et al. Thymectomy task force formed by the Medical Advisory Board of the Myasthenia Gravis Foundation of America. Ann Thorac Surg 1997;64:1311.
14. Jaretzki A III. Thymectomy for myasthenia gravis: analysis of the controversies regarding technique and results. Neurology 1997;48(suppl 5):S52-63.
15. Bedlack RS, Simel DL, Bosworth H, et al. Quantitative myasthenia gravis score: assessment of responsiveness and longitudinal validity. Neurology 2005; 64(11):1968-70.
16. Alshaikh JT, Amdur R, Sidawy A, et al. Thymectomy is safe for myasthenia gravis patients: analysis of the NSQIP database. Muscle Nerve 2016;53(3):370-4.
17. Lee CY, Kim DJ, Lee JG, et al. Bilateral video-assisted thoracoscopic thymectomy has a surgical extent similar to that of transsternal extended thymectomy with more favorable early surgical outcomes for myasthenia gravis patients. Surg Endosc 2011;25:849-54.
18. Shrager JB, Deeb ME, Mick R, et al. Transcervical thymectomy for myasthenia gravis achieves results comparable to thymectomy by sternotomy. Ann Thorac Surg 2002;74:320-7.
19. Mack MJ, Landreneau RJ, Yim AP, et al. Results of video-assisted thymectomy in patients with myasthenia gravis. J Thorac Cardiovasc Surg 1996;112: 1352-60.
20. Ponseti JM, Gamuz J, Vilallonga R, et al. Influence of ectopic thymic tissue on clinical outcome following extended thymectomy in generalized seropositive nonthymomatous myasthenia gravis. Eur J Cardiothorac Surg 2008;34:1062-7.
21. Miller RG, Filler-Katz A, Kiprov D, et al. Repeat thymectomy in chronic refractory myasthenia gravis. Neurology 1991;41:923-4.
22. Jaretzki A III, Penn AS, Younger DS, et al. "Maximal" thymectomy for myasthenia gravis: results. J Thorac Cardiovasc Surg 1988;95:747-57.
23. Masaoka A, Monden Y, Seike Y, et al. Reoperation after transcervical thymectomy for myasthenia gravis. J Thorac Cardiovasc Surg 1982;32:83-5.
24. Wolfe GI, Kaminski HJ, Cutter GN. Randomized trial of thymectomy in myasthenia gravis. N Engl J Med 2016;375:2006-7.
25. Alshekhlee A, Miles JD, Katirji B, et al. Incidence and mortality rates of myasthenia gravis and myasthenic crisis in US hospitals. Neurology 2009;72: 1548-54.
26. Gilhus NE. Myasthenia gravis. N Engl J Med 2016; 375:2570-81.

27. Conti-Fine BM, Diethelm-Okita B, Ostlie N, et al. Immunopathogenesis of myasthenia gravis. In: Kaminski HJ, editor. Myasthenia gravis and related disorders. New York: Humana Press; 2009. p. 43–70.

28. Drachman DB. Myasthenia gravis. N Engl J Med 1994;330:1797–810.

29. Gilhus NE, Skeie GO, Romi F, et al. Myasthenia gravis - autoantibody characteristics and their implications for therapy. Nat Rev Neurol 2016;12(5): 259–68.

30. Weis C-A, Aban IB, Cutter G, et al. Histopathology of thymectomy specimens from the MGTX-trial: Entropy analysis as strategy to quantify spatial heterogeneity of lymphoid follicle and fat distribution. PLoS One 2018;13:e0197435.

31. Muscle Study Group. A trial of mycophenolate mofetil with prednisone as initial immunotherapy in myasthenia gravis. Neurology 2008;71:394–9.

32. Sanders DB, Hart IK, Mantegazza R, et al. An international, phase III, randomized trial of mycophenolate mofetil in myasthenia gravis. Neurology 2008; 71:400–6.

33. Gilhus NE. Myasthenia and the neuromuscular junction. Curr Opin Neurol 2012;25(5):523–9.

34. Verschuuren JJ, Huijbers MG, Plomp JJ, et al. Pathophysiology of myasthenia gravis with antibodies to the acetylcholine receptor, muscle-specific kinase and low-density lipoprotein receptor-related protein 4. Autoimmun Rev 2013;12(9):918–23.

35. Skeie GO, Apostolski S, Evoli A, et al. Guidelines for treatment of autoimmune neuromuscular transmission disorders. Eur J Neurol 2010;17(7):893–902.

36. Sanders DB, Wolfe GI, Benatar M, et al. International consensus guidance for the management of myasthenia gravis. Neurology 2016;87:419–25.

37. Roberts PF, Venuta F, Rendina E, et al. Thymectomy in the treatment of ocular myasthenia gravis. J Thorac Cardiovasc Surg 2001;122(3):562–8.

38. Schumm F, Wietholter H, Fateh-Moghadam A, et al. Thymectomy in myasthenia with pure ocular symptoms. J Neurol Neurosurg Psychiatry 1985;48(4): 332–7.

39. Papatestas AE, Genkins G, Kornfeld P, et al. Effects of thymectomy in myasthenia gravis. Ann Surg 1987; 206(1):79–88.

40. Hatton PD, Diehl JT, Daly BD, et al. Transsternal radical thymectomy for myasthenia gravis: a 15-year review. Ann Thorac Surg 1989;47(6):838–40.

41. Masaoka A, Yamakawa Y, Niwa H, et al. Extended thymectomy for myasthenia gravis patients: a 20-year review. Ann Thorac Surg 1996;62(3):853–9.

42. Nakamura H, Taniguchi Y, Suzuki Y, et al. Delayed remission after thymectomy for myasthenia gravis of the purely ocular type. J Thorac Cardiovasc Surg 1996;112(2):371–5.

History of Thymectomy for Myasthenia Gravis

Joel D. Cooper, MD

KEYWORDS

- Myasthenia gravis • History of thymectomy • Surgical management of myasthenia gravis
- Thymoma • Thymus • Transcervical • Myasthenic

KEY POINTS

- In the early 1900s, chance observations that incidental thymectomy performed in the course of thyroidectomy in several patients having both Graves' disease and myasthenia first suggested a relationship between myasthenia and the thymus gland.
- Autopsy findings or either a thymoma or thymic hypertrophy in patients dying of myasthenia gravis further suggested a relationship between the thymus gland and myasthenia.
- The similarity of symptoms between myasthenia gravis and curare poisoning pointed to the possibility of a defect in neuromuscular transmission.
- The discovery of acetylcholine as the transmitter for voluntary muscles resulted in the development of anticholinesterase drugs for the treatment of myasthenia and the use of the intravenous Tensilon injection test for diagnosis.
- Alfred Blalock's 1939 report of dramatic improvement in following excision of a thymic tumor in a myasthenic patient prompted further explanation of the role of thymectomy for this condition.
- From the middle of the past century to the present time, dramatic progress in the medical and surgical management of myasthenia gravis has greatly expanded the role of thymectomy for the management of this disease.

Myasthenia gravis is a neuromuscular disease characterized by weakness and fatigability of the voluntary muscles. Clinically, the onset of symptoms may be insidious or acute and may be manifested by weakness of the proximal limb muscles, ocular muscles, or bulbar muscles.

The clinical disorder now known as myasthenia gravis was described in 1877 by Wilks,[1] who reported a patient presenting with progressive weakness that ultimately resulted in death from respiratory paralysis. Over the next several years, similar case reports appeared in the literature. In 1893, Goldflam[2] summarized previously reported cases along with his own experience. He described the clinical findings that became known as Erb-Goldflam symptom-complex. The condition was later termed myasthenia gravis pseudoparalytica by Jolly and Ueber,[3] who described the classic decremental response to repetitive muscle stimulation in such patients.

The course of the disease may be indolent or progressive, may involve ocular, bulbar, or generalized distribution, and symptoms usually worsen with activity and improve with rest. The variability of symptoms and their severity, even from day to day, has often resulted in their being attributed to an emotional or psychiatric origin.

The pathophysiology of myasthenia gravis remained relatively obscure for more than 100 years. The similarity between the symptoms of myasthenia and those of curare poisoning suggested that myasthenia symptoms might be

Disclosure: The author has nothing to disclose.
Department of Surgery, Hospital of the University of Pennsylvania, 3400 Spruce Street, 6 White, Philadelphia, PA 19104, USA
E-mail address: Joel.cooper@uphs.upenn.edu

Thorac Surg Clin 29 (2019) 151–158
https://doi.org/10.1016/j.thorsurg.2018.12.011

related to blockade of transmission across the neuromuscular junction. The identification of acetylcholine as the neuromuscular transmitter released at voluntary motor nerve endings and the discovery that many patients with myasthenic symptoms had immediate, temporary improvement following the intravenous injection of anticholinesterase drugs, such as physostigmine,[4,5] further suggested that the neuromuscular junction was the site of the defect.

Myasthenia gravis is now recognized to represent an autoimmune disease resulting in reduction of the available acetylcholine receptor sites at the neuromuscular junction resulting from the presence of circulating autoimmune antibodies that bind to these sites. It remains uncertain as to what causes or triggers the autoimmune response.

Early observations of the possible benefit of thymectomy in patients with myasthenia gravis were in fact serendipitous, as the partial or complete resection of the thymus gland in such cases was performed in conjunction with simultaneous or staged operation on the adjacent enlarged thyroid gland (Graves' disease) for upper airway obstruction. Thus, in 1910, Garré removed an enlarged thymus from such a patient (a 22-year-old woman) and the symptoms of myasthenia were relieved.[6] In 1911, Ferdinand Sauerbruch removed the thymus gland as the first of a 2-stage procedure in a patient with Graves' disease accompanied by signs of myasthenia gravis. The second stage, a partial thyroidectomy, was done at a later date, but following the thymectomy stage, the patient's myasthenic symptoms greatly improved.[7]

It is of interest that the surgical approach used by Sauerbruch was the transcervical approach, used in those days in infants and young children with radiologic evidence of an enlarged large thymus gland believed to be the cause of upper respiratory symptoms or unexplained sudden death. Both operations were directed at relieving respiratory distress, thought to be related to compression of the airway in the cervical region.

In 1913, Charles Parker,[8] from Chicago, reported a case of thymectomy in a 1-year-old child who had recently presented with the onset of 2 to 3 convulsions a day associated with episodes of cyanosis. A successful thymectomy was performed for presumed upper airway obstruction caused by a hypertrophied thymus as was demonstrated on chest radiograph. Together with this case, he reviewed the literature and reported on 49 other cases of thymectomy, both published and unpublished, which he collected from the period beginning 1896 through April 1912.[8] His review indicated that most of the operations were directed toward the "relief of tracheal and esophageal obstruction due to hypertrophy of the gland, the not infrequent cause of sudden death in infants." He was able to find only 1 report of a thymectomy performed on an adult, this being the previously noted case performed by Garré,[6] which involved a 2-stage procedure for relief of airway obstruction in a patient with Graves' disease, with the first stage being a thymectomy and the second later stage being thyroidectomy.

The concept of surgical resection of the thymus gland, specifically for the treatment of myasthenia gravis, has its origins in reports by Weigert[9] and Bell,[10] who noted the prevalence of thymic abnormalities (hyperplasia, tumors) in autopsy findings in 75% of patients who had died of myasthenia gravis.

In May 1936, Dr. Alfred Blalock resected a tumor of the thymus gland in a 21-year old woman with symptoms of myasthenia gravis that had first appeared at age 16. The patient subsequently had recurrent episodes of exacerbation and partial remission. A chest radiograph revealed a sharply circumscribed, dense, anterior mediastinal mass extending to the left of the midline. The patient had a course of radiotherapy with diminution in the size of the mass. A second course of radiotherapy was administered several months later. A year afterward, the patient had another severe relapse and repeat radiograph showed enlargement of the tumor mass. The patient's symptoms responded to physostigmine, which had recently been shown to produce dramatic improvement in myasthenic symptoms. However, the patient's symptoms responded to such injections with diminishing benefit, and 4 more radiation treatments were administered without apparent shrinkage of the tumor but with gradual improvement of symptoms. After consultation with other prominent surgeons of his day, Dr. Blalock proceeded with resection of the tumor through an upper partial midline sternotomy. On pathologic examination, the patient's mass proved to be a well-encapsulated benign cystic tumor, presumably of thymic origin. The patient showed steady improvement and a preliminary report was published the following year.[11] Three years later, Dr. Blalock reported that the patient, "who had been incapacitated for months every year for 4 years prior to the operation has had only one mild recurrence which lasted only few days, associated with a severe respiratory infection."[12] He noted that she almost certainly would have died had prostigmin not just become available for preoperative and perioperative management of her myasthenic symptoms. In his report, Blalock reviewed the clinical and experimental evidence accumulated to date, indicating a probable relationship between the thymus gland and myasthenia gravis. He also reviewed all available reports of the anatomic description of the thymus gland in patients with myasthenia gravis, either at postmortem examination or at operation. Approximately half of all the reports, demonstrated abnormalities either in the form of tumor or hyperplasia. On the basis of his review, and his experience with his own previously reported patient, Blalock concluded that the evidence might indicate, "the advisability of the surgical removal of clinically demonstrable thymic tumors in patients with myasthenia gravis."

In 1941, Blalock embarked on a clinical trial with the intention of completely removing all thymus tissue in patients with myasthenia gravis either with or without evidence of a tumor, in hopes of altering the course of the disease. He reported the preliminary results in 6 such patients on whom he had recently done a median sternotomy for this purpose.[13] All patients had severe symptoms, 5 being generalized and 1 being ocular and bulbar only. None of the patients had an apparent tumor, and all were prepared for surgery with a preoperative course of the recently available prostigmin bromide. Final pathology showed persistent thymic tissue in all 6 of the patients, 5 with definite hyperplasia. There was 1 postoperative death, in the patient with severe preoperative bulbar symptoms who died of aspiration pneumonia. Clinical follow-up at 2 to 3 months postoperative showed that 3 patients had marked improvement or remission of symptoms and the 2 remaining patients had benefit of a lesser degree.

Blalock's[13] report stimulated considerable interest in the use of thymectomy for the treatment of myasthenia gravis over the ensuing 20 years. However, in patients without a thymoma, it was used with great caution, and generally in younger patients with moderate to severe disease, whose symptoms were refractory to medical treatment.

In 1966, a landmark report was published representing a cooperative study between the myasthenia gravis clinic at the Massachusetts General Hospital (MGH) established in 1935, and the Mt. Sinai Hospital myasthenia gravis clinic in New York established in 1951.[14] This study, which included 1355 patients, represented an attempt to evaluate the relative effectiveness of medical and surgical treatment and to clarify the role of thymectomy in the treatment of myasthenia gravis. Thymectomy, in selected cases, had been used at MGH since 1941 and at the Mt. Sinai Hospital since 1951. Of the 1013 patients surviving at the time of the report, 50% had been followed from 5 to 15 years and 25% for more than 15 years. The demographics of the patients at the 2 centers were quite similar in terms of the sex and age at onset of symptoms and consistent with previous reports. Sixty percent were women and 40% were men. Importantly, two-thirds of female patients had the onset of symptoms when younger than the age of 40, whereas as two-thirds of the male patients had the onset of symptoms when older than 40.

The severity of disease at onset and at follow-up was determined using a modified Osserman classification, shown in **Table 1**.

For follow-up evaluation, the same clinical classification was used, with the addition of group "A" to indicate complete remission following treatment.

In the combined MGH-Mt. Sinai series, use of thymectomy in patients without a thymoma was generally reserved for patients younger than 40, with moderate to severe symptoms refractory to medical management. There were 186 such patients, only 30 of whom were men because, as the previously noted age and sex distribution indicates, and selection criteria, greatly favored women. The results of thymectomy in the female group showed striking benefit with a 38% total remission rate and an additional 51% improvement rate. For nonoperated women, the complete remission rate was 14%, with an additional 18% improved. Ninety-two percent of patients in the operated group had symptoms classified as 2B or higher, whereas only 35% of the nonoperated patients had symptoms in this range. In the operated group, the most recent follow-up showed a 37% complete remission rate with an additional 55% showing improvement. In the nonoperated patients with the same preoperative moderate to severe initial status, 8% achieved remission, 49% were improved, 41% were unchanged, and 2% were worse. Results in the male population were also encouraging, but the experience with

Table 1 Modified Osserman classification of symptoms	
Group 1	Ocular involvement only
Group 2A	Mild, generalized symptoms including ocular involvement
Group 2B	Moderately severe generalized symptoms including ocular and mild bulbar involvement
Group 3	Acute, severe symptoms developing over a period of weeks to months with severe bulbar involvement
Group 4	Late, severe, progressive with bulbar involvement

such patients was considered too limited to derive definitive conclusions.

In the overall group of patients with myasthenia gravis in the MGH/Mt. Sinai report, there were 129 patients who had thymoma, most of whom did not undergo operation. The prognosis for the overall group was poor and the role of thymectomy for such patients remained uncertain. However, for myasthenic patients without a thymoma, the report concluded that, "operation is recommended for females under 40 years of age who have severe, generalized myasthenia which does not respond satisfactory to drug or x-ray therapy. The value of thymectomy for females over age 40 is less certain. The role of thymectomy in males is still uncertain on statistical grounds although operation does seem indicated for selected male patients." The report also concluded that, "for myasthenic patients with thymomas, a combination of x-ray treatments and operation is indicated, despite generally poor prognosis for these patients." The poor prognosis for such patients related more to the thymoma than to the myasthenia, as the thymoma in such patients was often discovered at a late stage. With the advent of computed tomography scans, and the practice of obtaining one when the diagnosis of myasthenia is made, associated thymomas are found at a much earlier stage.

As previously noted, the earliest reports of thymectomy, at the beginning of the twentieth century, were performed through a transcervical approach when it was thought that thymic enlargement in infants was a common cause of respiratory symptoms due to airway compression at the thoracic inlet. However, following Blalock's report,[13] the cervical approach was generally abandoned in favor of median sternotomy. However, there was considerable morbidity and mortality associated with this approach given that most patients had severe myasthenic symptoms at the time of operation, including respiratory compromise, at a time when there were limited options for medical management, and when anesthetic management, use of postoperative ventilatory assistance, and respiratory care in general, were relatively primitive by today's standards.

In the 267 nonthymoma patients undergoing thymectomy for myasthenia gravis reported in the MGH/Mt. Sinai series, there are no details regarding operative mortality or morbidity. The median sternotomy approach was used in 239 patients. In the remaining 28 patients, the use of a transcervical thymectomy was reintroduced by Dr. Kirschner, at the Mt. Sinai Hospital toward the end of the series, in hopes of simplifying and improving the postoperative course and reducing the risk. In 1969, Kirschner and colleagues[15] reported subsequent experience with this technique in 21 consecutive patients over the preceding 2 years. In this series, patients with radiologic evidence of a thymoma were generally excluded except for 2 patients with a very small, well-circumscribed tumor.

Kirschner and colleagues[15] reported that with the use of the transcervical approach, the postoperative course was simplified and the risk of mortality and morbidity were reduced. Accordingly, the indications for patient selection were liberalized to include patients with milder forms of the disease and shorter duration of symptoms. Even so, a tracheostomy was performed at the end of the procedure in all patients without an existing tracheostomy. The almost complete absence of pain and discomfort following the procedure allowed for increased mobility and early ambulation with only limited and infrequent doses of analgesia required. Otherwise, however, the postoperative management protocol was similar to that used for transsternal thymectomy, including avoidance, as much as possible, of any cholinergic drugs, for the first 5 days followed by cautious introduction of cholinergic medication whose need was confirmed by repeated Tensilon testing. Ventilator assistance was provided through the tracheostomy tube as clinically indicated.

In the series of 21 transcervical thymectomies reported by Kirschner and colleagues,[15] there was 1 postoperative death. One-year follow-up was available for 12 patients, 3 of whom had "border-line" complete remission, 6 showed improvement, and 3 showed no change. For the remaining 8 remaining patients, the follow-up period was too short to evaluate the effect of the operation. It was acknowledged that there was insufficient evidence to indicate whether or not the long-term results with this approach would be equivalent to those following the standard sternotomy approach, but the reduced morbidity and mortality alone were sufficient for, Kirschner and colleagues[15] to conclude that "the transcervical total thymectomy is now our surgical procedure of choice in myasthenia gravis."

From the mid-1960s through the 1970s, thymectomy was increasingly but not universally used in the management of myasthenia gravis. Although no randomized trial between medical and surgical therapy had been conducted, the value of thymectomy in the long-term management of myasthenia was strongly supported by the report of Buckingham and colleagues[16] from the Mayo Clinic in 1967. This study compared the long-term outcome of patients undergoing thymectomy for myasthenia gravis with computer-assisted matching of these patients to a similar group of patients, in terms of severity and medical management, but who did not undergo thymectomy. The results demonstrated that the thymectomized patients had a significantly higher rate of complete remission and improved long-term survival, in comparison with those receiving medical therapy alone.

In 1974, Mulder and coworkers[17] at the UCLA Medical Center reported their experience in 100 consecutive patients undergoing thymectomy with careful follow-up studies up to 16 years. These patients were selected from the 443 patients with confirmed myasthenia gravis seen at their institution during the same time period. Transsternal thymectomy was performed as an elective procedure and "never during an acute relapse or myasthenic crisis." This series included patients with or without thymoma, but patients without a thymoma and having only mild symptoms that were readily controlled with anticholinesterase drugs were excluded.

In 50 of the 100 patients, concomitant tracheostomy was performed at the time of thymectomy specifically on those patients with bulbar symptoms, previous respiratory complications, a history of previous myasthenic complications, or a vital capacity of less than 2 L. In all other patients, a naso-tracheal tube was left in place to facilitate postoperative respiratory management, and eliminate the need for anticholinesterase therapy in the early postoperative period because of the previously noted difficulty in differentiating symptoms of insufficient doses of medication from those of toxic doses. In 6 of the 50 patients left with a tracheal tube in place postoperatively, only 6 required conversion to a tracheostomy within the first 48 hours after operation, thus sparing 44 patients a tracheostomy, which was still routinely used in all patients undergoing thymectomy at many centers. There were 2 postoperative deaths in this series, reflecting the ongoing progress achieved in the preoperative and postoperative management of these patients.

In 1978, Drachman[18,19] published a 2-part report in the New England Journal of Medicine, comprehensively summarizing the current knowledge as to the pathophysiology of myasthenia gravis and its treatment. Drachman's review[18,19] acknowledged the potentially beneficial effects of thymectomy as confirmed by published results of a large series of surgically treated cases that demonstrated improvement in 57% to 86% of patients. He also noted that there remained many unanswered questions, including the indications for thymectomy, the optimal surgical approach, and the absence of definitive prognostic factors as to the likely outcome in individual patients.

With improvements in medical and surgical management of myasthenic patients, the refinement in techniques to diagnose myasthenia gravis earlier in the course of the disease, and the perception that thymectomy early in the course of the disease produced the optimum result, utilization of thymectomy as part of the overall treatment for myasthenia gravis became more widespread, the indications less strict, and upper age limits less rigid.

Two anatomic studies have demonstrated the widespread variance in the distribution of thymic tissue in the cervical and anterior mediastinal region, including occasional microscopic foci in adjacent fat.[20,21] However, the goal of accomplishing such a radical excision not only of all visible thymic and perithymic tissue but also of any possible remote unrecognizable microscopic foci, as the standard approach for thymectomy in myasthenic patients, requires a full sternotomy along with concomitant cervical exploration. Such a radical approach, however, conflicts with the increasing utilization of thymectomy early in the course of the disease, even in patients with minimum, well-controlled symptoms under medical management. For such patients, and their neurologists, the prospect of undergoing such a procedure poses a significant barrier to incorporating thymectomy as part of the long-term strategy, especially when the cause of the disease is unpredictable and the benefit of the procedure for any individual patient is uncertain.

As previously noted, the use of a transcervical approach for thymectomy was reintroduced by Kirschner and colleagues[15] primarily in an attempt to reduce the significant morbidity and mortality associated with the sternotomy approach in those days. The transcervical approach was subsequently adopted at other centers including at The University of Toronto, where Cooper and colleagues[22] in 1988 reported a modified technique using a self-retaining retractor to elevate the manubrium. This facilitated direct visualization and improved access to the entire thymus gland and perithymic fatty tissue through a small cervical excision. This report also presented results of 65 consecutive myasthenic patients without thymoma undergoing transcervical thymectomy over the preceding 8 years. There was no postoperative mortality or significant complication, no necessity for intraoperative conversion to sternotomy, no need for tracheostomy or ventilator assistance beyond a matter of hours spent in the recovery room, and no blood transfusion requirement. Ninety percent of patients were discharged within 48 hours. All patients were followed for a minimum of 1 year (median, 3.5 years). There was no mortality within the first 4 years of follow-up (with 2 later unrelated deaths).

Importantly, the results in the Toronto report were compared with those reported using a standard sternotomy approach, at Duke University[23] and with the results reported by Jaretzki and colleagues[24] at Columbia University, using the combined sternotomy and cervical approach for a radical excision of all thymic tissue and adjacent fatty tissues. Five-year follow-up of each report showed virtually identical results, in terms of percentage of patients with complete remission, percentage of patients asymptomatic with minimal medication, and percentage of patients showing no apparent improvement.

The essentially equivalent results from these 3 series might be cited as evidence that even the most complete possible thymectomy, as proposed by Jaretzki,[24] does not result in a complete remission in half or more of the patients. This suggests that complete thymectomy alone is not the overall solution for the management of myasthenia gravis. Alternatively, one might argue that because 3 different surgical approaches all gave essentially the same results, the clinical improvement over time following thymectomy had little if anything to do with the thymectomy and more to do with the various medical protocols used, and the unpredictable natural course of myasthenia gravis.

In 1997, Jaretzki[25] published a very complete review of the literature (with 123 references) together with a thoughtful analysis of the persisting controversies regarding the role of surgical resection and an analysis of the results reported with each of the differing surgical techniques. He noted that at least 7 different surgical procedures had been used, at least 8 different classifications for describing the severity of symptoms were reported, and there was no consistent method for analyzing the outcomes following surgical resection. He concluded that, "the thymectomy literature is replete with confusing data, variously defined measurements and unsupported conclusions." He called for the development of a uniform classification of severity symptoms, a clearly predefined measure of success, and the use of such measures to compare thymectomy techniques. His review included illustrations of the variations in the anatomy of the thymus gland, based on the surgical anatomy in 50 consecutive operations using the combined transcervical and transsternal "maximal" thymectomy approach that he had previously published,[26] and expressed his belief that "the more aggressive the resection, the higher the remission rate."

A follow-up to the University of Toronto experience with transcervical thymectomy was reported in 1999, and reviewed results with the most recent 100 consecutive cases for nonthymoma-associated myasthenia gravis between 1989 to 1998.[27] Median follow-up was 5.3 years. This report highlighted the more liberal application of thymectomy compared with the original series of 65 patients reported more than 10 years earlier. In the most recent series, the patients were an average of 11 years older than in the initial series (38 vs 27), and included a higher percentage of patients who were receiving prednisone at the time of operation (33% vs 11%). There was no operative mortality, no serious complication, a mean hospital stay of 1.2 days, and with 90% of patients being discharged on the first postoperative day. Patients reported ability to return to unrestricted complete activity within 5 days.

The difficulty in comparing the 2 series was also noted, due to interim changes in the long-term medical management of patients. In the initial report, complete remission was defined as patients with no symptoms and no requirement for medication. At the time of the second report, however, it had been common for such patients to be maintained on low-dose immunosuppression, such as alternate-day prednisone or other agent, which was thought to reduce the risk of reemergence of symptoms. This is often referred to as "pharmacologic" remission. Thus, even the most objective of outcomes, complete remission, could not be used to compare results in the 2 reports, as this definition could not be applied in the same fashion to both series. The 5-year complete remission rate in the first series was 52% versus a rate of 46% having "pharmacologic" remission at 5 years in the second series.

Over the past 50 years, very significant advances have been made in the understanding of the pathophysiology of myasthenia gravis as an autoimmune disease and correspondingly in its medical management. This includes the introduction of plasmapheresis, which, along with prednisone and aziathioprine, was shown to produce striking immediate clinical improvement in patients, with myasthenia gravis having persistent moderate to severe disability despite high-dose prednisone therapy and optimal doses of cholinesterase inhibitors.[28] The use of plasmapheresis and/or the administration of intravenous immunoglobulin to produce rapid, short-term improvement in muscle weakness has been of particular value in optimizing patients' symptoms before thymectomy, and permit rapid tapering of the prednisone dose in anticipation of surgery, to further reduce the risk of complications.

Despite the increasing acceptance of the overall benefit of thymectomy in general, the relatively low risk and minimal morbidity now associated with the procedure, and observations that the earlier in the course of disease it is used the sooner and more durable the benefit,[29,30] there remains uncertainty as to which patients might benefit. Thus thymectomy for nonthymoma patients has become essentially a "test of surgery," with prospective patients advised that benefit is uncertain and might not be manifest for 5 years or more. This in turn has placed increased emphasis on the use of minimally invasive surgical techniques, including transcervical, video-assisted, and robotic-assisted approaches to reduce morbidity as much as possible, and foster acceptability of thymectomy as part of the long-term management strategy for this disease.

In the absence of a randomized trial, the Quality Standards Subcommittee of the American Academy of Neurology reported in 2000 a systematic review of the literature,[31] and concluded that the available evidence supported the use of thymectomy as an option to improve outcome and noted that further studies, and ideally randomized controlled trials, should be pursued.

In 2013, a Cochrane Database review of relevant published reports[32] concluded that there was inadequate scientific evidence with which to validate the benefit of thymectomy in nonthymomatous patients with myasthenia gravis, and concluded that randomized and "quasi-randomized" studies were needed.

In 2016, the long-awaited results of a randomized trial evaluating the benefit of thymectomy was reported by the Myasthenia Gravis Thymectomy Trial Study Group in the *New England Journal of Medicine*.[33]

This trial mandated a highly specific, medical management protocol for all patients, which required the use of alternate day prednisone as the primary medication, with frequent monitoring and adjustment of the dose to achieve "minimal manifestation status." Patients were then randomized to either the addition of thymectomy or no thymectomy. The thymectomy required full median sternotomy and "extended" excision of all thymus tissue and adjacent fat from the cervical and mediastinal fields. Both groups were maintained on long-term alternating-day prednisone with adjustment of the dose to maintain minimal manifestation status if possible.

The trial was initiated in 2006, extended over 9 years, and included 36 international centers. It required the screening of 6958 patients with myasthenia, and 2 subsequent relaxations of eligibility criteria, to enroll the 126 patients who underwent randomization. Assessment of outcome was done using a time-weighted average of the quantitative scoring system used to evaluate symptoms (on a scale of 0–39) and a time-weighted average of the dose of prednisone required to achieve "a minimal manifestation status." Both of these scoring systems were averaged over a 3-year follow-up period. Recognizing the significant limitations of the trial, and the highly selective group of patients evaluated, it was concluded that patients who underwent thymectomy did have improved results compared with the control group, in terms of improvement of symptoms and in terms of the 3-year average dosage of alternate-day prednisone required to achieve the minimal manifestation status. However, the limited number of patients, the use of a very complex and labor-intensive method of evaluating the outcome, the absence of data regarding the achievement of complete remission or complete pharmacologic remission, the highly structured medication protocol using alternate-day prednisone, often of high doses, as the primary immunosuppression agent (without replacing prednisone with newer immunosuppressive agents), all but eliminate the possibility of comparing the results of this study with the results of other previous or future studies attempting to define the role of thymectomy in the treatment of myasthenia gravis. This much anticipated clinical trial may confirm the longstanding presumption that thymectomy does indeed have a significant role to play in the long-term management of myasthenia gravis, but its complexity and highly selective eligibility will also likely have a very chilling effect on any future proposals to embark on a randomized clinical trial seeking to better define the role of thymectomy for most patients with myasthenia or to confirm whether a radical surgical approach is superior to a less invasive one.

After more than a century since the first demonstration that thymectomy may be of value in the treatment of myasthenia gravis, controversy remains as to which patients to choose, when to consider it, what procedure to use, and how to evaluate its benefit. The answers to these questions remain the "holy grail."

REFERENCES

1. Wilks S. On cerebritis, hysteria and bulbar paralysis. Guys Hosp Rep 1877;22:7.
2. Goldflam S. Ueber einen scheinbar heilbaren bulbar paralytischen symptomen complex mit Beteiligung der Extremitaten. Dtsch Z Nervenheilkd 1893;4:312.
3. Jolly F. Ueber. Myasthenia gravis pseudoparalytica. Berl Klin Wochenschr 1895;32:1–7.

4. Walker MB. Treatment of myasthenia gravis with physostigmine. Lancet 1934;1:1200.

5. Walker MB. Case showing effect of prostigmine on myasthenia gravis. Proc R Soc Med 1935;28:759.

6. Capelle, Behr. Garré operator. Operative case. June 26, 1910. Beitr. X. kiln. Chir., Tübingen 1911;lxxii: 214.

7. Schumacher, Roth. Thymektomie bei einem Fall von Morbus Basedowii mit Myasthenia. Mitt a d Grenzgeb d Med u Chir 1912;25:746.

8. Parker CA. Surgery of the thymus gland. Thymectomy. Report of fifty operated cases. Amer Jour Dis Child 1913;5(2):89–122.

9. Weigert C. Pathologisch-anatomischer Beitrag zur Erb-schen Krankheit (Myasthenia Gravis). Neurol Zentralbl 1901;20:597–601.

10. Bell ET. Tumors of the thymus in myasthenia gravis. J Nerv Ment Dis 1917;45(130).

11. Riven SS, Mason MF. Southern Med Jour 1937;30: 181.

12. Blalock A, Mason MF, Morgan HJ, et al. Myasthenia gravis and tumors of thymic region. Ann Surg 1939; 4(110):544–61.

13. Blalock A, Harvey AM, Ford FR, et al. JAMA 1949; 117(18):1529–33.

14. Perlo VP, Schwab RS, Osserman KE. Myasthenia gravis: evaluation of treatment in 1,335 patients. Neurology 1965;5(16):431–9.

15. Kirschner PA, Osserman KE, Kark AE. Studies in myasthenia gravis: transcervical total thymectomy. JAMA 1969;209(6):906–10.

16. Buckingham JM, Howard FM, Bernatz PE, et al. The value of thymectomy in myasthenia gravis: a computer-assisted matched study. Ann Surg 1976; 184:453–8.

17. Mulder DG, Herrmann C, Buckberg GD. Effect of thymectomy in patients with myasthenia gravis. Am J Surg 1974;128:202–6.

18. Drachman DB. Myasthenia gravis (first of two parts). N Engl J Med 1978;298:136–42.

19. Drachman DB. Myasthenia gravis (second of two parts). N Engl J Med 1978;298:186–93.

20. Masaoka A, Nagaoka Y, Kotake Y. Distribution of thymic tissue at the anterior mediastinum: current procedures in thymectomy. J Thorac Cardiovasc Surg 1975;70(4):747–54.

21. Jaretzki A III, Bethea M, Wolff M, et al. A rational approach to total thymectomy in the treatment of myasthenia gravis. Ann Thorac Surg 1977;24(2): 120–30.

22. Cooper JD, Al-Jilaihawa AN, Pearson FG, et al. An improved technique to facilitate transcervical thymectomy for myasthenia gravis. Ann Thorac Surg 1988;45:242–7.

23. Olanow CW, Wechsler AS, Sirotkin-Roses M, et al. Thymectomy as primary therapy in myasthenia gravis. Ann N Y Acad Sci 1986;505:595.

24. Jaretzki A III, Penn AS, Younger DS, et al. "Maximal" thymectomy for myasthenia gravis: results. J Thorac Cardiovasc Surg 1988;95:747–57.

25. Jaretzki A III. Thymectomy for myasthenia gravis: analysis of the controversies regarding technique and results. Neurology 1997;48(suppl 5):S52–63.

26. Jaretzki A III, Wolf M. "Maximal" thymectomy for myasthenia gravis: surgical anatomy and operative technique. J Thorac Cardiovasc Surg 1988;96: 711–6.

27. Calhoun RF, Ritter JH, Guthrie RN, et al. Results of transcervical thymectomy for myasthenia gravis in 100 consecutive patients. Ann Surg 1999;230(4): 555–61.

28. Dau PC, Lindstrom JM, Cassel CK, et al. Plasmapheresis and immunosuppressive drug therapy in myasthenia gravis. N Engl J Med 1977;297: 1134–40.

29. Genkins G, Papatestas AE, Horowitz SH, et al. Studies in myasthenia gravis: early thymectomy. Am J Med 1975;58(4):517–24.

30. Maggi G, Casadio A, Cavallo CR. Thymectomy in myasthenia gravis: results of 662 cases operated upon in 15 years. Eur J Cardiothorac Surg 1989; 3(6):504–9.

31. Gronseth GSG, Barohn RJR. Practice parameter: thymectomy for autoimmune myasthenia gravis: an evidence-based review): report of the Quality Standards Subcommittee of the American Academy of Neurology. Neurology 2000;55(1):7–15.

32. Cea G, Benatar M, Verdugo RJ, et al. Thymectomy for non-thymomatous myasthenia gravis. Cochrane Database Syst Rev 2013;(10):CD008111.

33. Wolfe GI, Kaminski HJ, Aban IB, et al. Randomized trial of thymectomy in myasthenia gravis. N Engl J Med 2016;375(6):511–22.

Surgical Approaches to Myasthenia Gravis
Perspective of Anatomy and Radicality in Surgery

Marcin Zieliński, MD, PhD

KEYWORDS

- Thymectomy • Mediastinum • Thymus gland • Thoracic surgery • Video-assisted
- Myasthenia gravis

KEY POINTS

- Removal of the thymic tissue is beneficial for the clinical course of myasthenia gravis (MG). During thymectomy, a complete removal of the thymus gland is obligatory.
- Removal of the ectopic thymic foci increases the chance for achieving complete remission, or substantial improvement of MG.
- Minimally invasive thoracic procedures are those performed through the intercostal, subxiphoid, or transcervical incisions.
- The definition of an extended thymectomy is a removal of the whole thymus with the surrounding adipose tissue that might contain the ectopic thymic foci.
- Minimally invasive technique of thymectomy should as extensive as the transsternal extended one.

INTRODUCTION

Historically, the first known thymectomy was reported in 1912 by Sauerbruch, the father of thoracic surgery who performed a transcervical subtotal thyroidectomy with concomitant subtotal thymectomy on a patient suffering from myasthenia gravis (MG) and hyperthyroidism with subsequent clinical improvement of MG and no improvement of hyperthyroidismus.[1] The surgeon who deliberately started to perform thymectomy for MG was Blalock,[1] who reported in 1939 a series of cases operated on through the median sternotomy approach with mixed results in terms of treatment of MG. Because of excessive operative risk of transsternal thymectomy, in that time the transcervical approach was re-introduced by several surgeons from 1965.[2] This technique was especially championed by Papatestas and colleagues,[3] who reported on the impressive number of almost 1000 patients operated on with the transcervical technique. Papatestas[3] declared openly that the procedure he performed was only a subtotal thymectomy and explained that, in his opinion, there was no need to do a total thymectomy for MG, similarly as there was no need for total thyroidectomy for the treatment of hyperthyroidism. With the elapse of time it became clear that there were many patients with a recurrent MG after these incomplete operations, and the recurrence was caused by a part of the thymus left behind in the mediastinum.[4,5] The fundamental studies, explaining the role of complete resection of the thymus and, what is even more important, discovery of the value of removal of the ectopic foci of the thymic tissue dispersed in the adipose tissue of the fat and the mediastinum were made by Masaoka and colleagues[6] and Jaretzki and Wolff.[7] Based on the detailed anatomic postmortem studies, Jaretzki and Wolff[7] found the ectopic

Disclosure: The author has nothing to disclose.
Department of the Thoracic Surgery, Pulmonary Hospital, Ul. Gładkie 1, Zakopane 34 500, Poland
E-mail address: marcinz@mp.pl

thoracic.theclinics.com

thymic foci in various locations in the neck, around the thyroid. Most of the investigators agreed in that time, that thymectomy for nonthymomatous MG should be performed in the transsternal extended technique. However, the 1990s brought some significant changes. First, the new minimally invasive techniques of thymectomy were introduced, including video-thoracoscopic (VATS) thymectomy and transcervical extended thymectomy.[8,9] In addition, the introduction of evidence-based medicine (EBM) led to reevaluation of many surgical techniques, including thymectomy for nonthymomatous MG.[10] The use of EBM challenged the previously accepted view of the beneficial role of thymectomy in the treatment of MG, which was based on the retrospective studies.[11] According to the EBM methodology, for the past several decades, until recently, the problem of superiority of operative treatment of MG over conservative treatment has not been solved unequivocally. It has been pointed out that there were no prospective randomized trials confirming better results of thymectomy versus medical treatment of MG. This changed in 2016, when the publication of the results of the international prospective randomized trial showed clearly that the results of patients who underwent a transsternal extended thymectomy and steroid therapy were significantly better, in comparison with patients treated with steroids alone.[12] What do we currently know about the value of thymectomy for MG? Thanks to the publication of the study of Wolfe and colleagues[12] there is no doubt that removal of the thymic tissue is beneficial for the clinical course of MG. During thymectomy, a complete removal of the thymus gland is obligatory. However, a necessity of performance of so-called extended thymectomy, with complete resection of the thymus supplemented by removal of the surrounding adipose tissue of the anterior mediastinum and the lower neck, is still a matter of controversy.

The results of several retrospective studies suggested that a removal of the ectopic thymic foci was also beneficial and increased the chance for achieving complete remission, or substantial improvement of MG.[13,14]

There have been enough data accumulated over time to assume that the way thymectomy is performed should be as radical as possible. Jaretzki and Wolff[7] distinguished several areas of the neck and mediastinum that should be explored during an operation to remove the fatty tissue that might contain the ectopic thymic foci. At my institution, we introduced a modified and simplified scheme of the areas of the adipose tissue necessary to remove during an extended or maximally extended thymectomy.[14] The aim of this article was to describe in detail how in our opinion an extended thymectomy for a patient with nonthymomatous MG should be performed.

RESULTS

We distinguish 6 areas of the adipose tissue surrounding the thymus gland (**Fig. 1**) including the following.

1. The lower neck, around and below the thyroid gland, down to the thoracic outlet level. Our definition differs from that of Jaretzki and Wolff,[7] who described the thymic foci above and behind the thyroid. To reach and remove such foci, it is necessary to perform an additional cervicotomy in every patient undergoing thymectomy, which is rarely practiced during the use of VATS techniques. In addition, it would be necessary to dissect both lobes of the thyroid gland to reach the area behind the thyroid, where the ectopic foci could be found (incidence 6% in the study of Jaretzki and Wolff,[7] and 9% in the study of Mizia and colleagues[15]). Such maneuvers would increase the risk of injury of the laryngeal recurrent nerves. Our institutional practice is to remove the whole tissue located below the lower poles of the thyroid lobes. This policy is based on the finding that we never found any ectopic foci

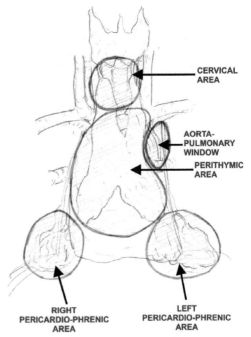

Fig. 1. The areas of ectopic foci of the thymic tissue that should be dissected during an extended thymectomy.

located higher in the neck than the previously mentioned level of the lower poles of the thyroid. We never dissected behind the thyroid. After dissection of the tissue below the thyroid, the lower poles of the thyroid, the innominate artery, both common carotid arteries, and the trachea should be clearly visible. In case we use the transcervical-subxiphoid-bilateral VATS approach, we additionally visualize both vagus and laryngeal recurrent nerves and the internal jugular veins bilaterally. We omit dissection of these structures if we use the subxiphoid-VATS approach, without a cervicotomy.

2. The perithymic area. The perithymic area is probably adequately dissected on most of minimally invasive techniques of thymectomy. The dissection should include complete removal of the tissue from one phrenic nerve to the other and from the left innominate vein (upper border), down to the diaphragm and removal of both epiphrenic fat pads, the aorta-caval groove, including the right paratracheal space.

3. The term aovta-caval groove was introduced by Jaretzki and Wolff,[7] but at our institution we changed its meaning and regarded this location as a space located between the ascending aorta and the superior vena cava, including the right paratracheal space.[7,14] The aorta-caval groove is a space contained between the innominate artery and the right subclavian artery (upper border), the right wall of the ascending aorta and the trachea (medial border), the right mediastinal pleura (lateral border), and the right main bronchus and the azygos vein (lower border) (**Fig. 2**). The incidence of the

ectopic foci in this location was 17.2%, according to our institutional data.[14] This area is beyond the reach for the left VATS approach, but it is possible to remove the content of this with use of the median sternotomy, right VATS, subxiphoid, and transcervical techniques.

4. The aorta-pulmonary window: the space between the left side of the ascending aorta, the left pulmonary artery and the left mediastinal pleura (**Fig. 3**).

    This is an especially important area with an incidence of ectopic foci of 25.9% and should be always dissected in case of nonthymomatous MG and thymoma-associated MG. This space is contained between the left wall of the ascending aorta (medial border),and the left pulmonary artery (lower border). The lateral and anterior border is made by the left mediastinal pleura with a left phrenic nerve. After dissection of the content of this space, the left vagus nerve should be visible and is a marker of an adequate completeness of dissection. A complete removal of the aorta-pulmonary window content is hardly possible from the right VATS approach.

5. The right pericardio-phrenic fat: the fatty tissue below the lower poles of the thymus including the right epiphrenic fat pad. It adheres to the right lower part of the pericardium and the right dome of the diaphragm. To resect the right epiphrenic it is important to avoid injury of the right phrenic nerve, so during dissection the nerve must be constantly visible. Therefore, it is impossible to resect the right epiphrenic from the left

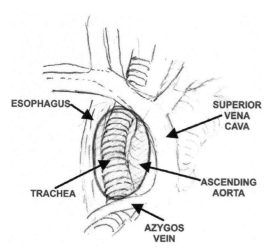

ESOPHAGUS
SUPERIOR VENA CAVA
TRACHEA
ASCENDING AORTA
AZYGOS VEIN

Fig. 2. The aorta-caval groove including the right paratracheal space.

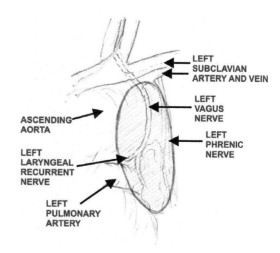

LEFT SUBCLAVIAN ARTERY AND VEIN
LEFT VAGUS NERVE
ASCENDING AORTA
LEFT PHRENIC NERVE
LEFT LARYNGEAL RECURRENT NERVE
LEFT PULMONARY ARTERY

Fig. 3. The aorta-pulmonary window.

VATS approach and it would be very difficult to do that through the transcervical approach. The right pericardio-phrenic area might contain the ectopic foci with an incidence of approximately 10%.

6. The left pericardio-phrenic fat: the fatty tissue below the lower poles of the thymus including the left epiphrenic fat pad. It adheres to the left lower part of the pericardium and the left dome of the diaphragm. To resect the left epiphrenic, it is important to avoid injury of the left phrenic nerve, so during dissection the nerve must be constantly visible. Therefore, it is impossible to resect the left epiphrenic from the right VATS approach and it would be very difficult to do that through the transcervical approach. The left pericardio-phrenic area might contain the ectopic foci with an incidence of approximately 10%. According to the results of Mizia and colleagues,[15] no ectopic foci were found in the epiphrenic fat pads, so the necessity of removal of this most caudal part of the pericardio-phrenic is not proven.

DISCUSSION

The meaning of finding of the ectopic foci and their removal for the therapeutic effects is ambiguous. The results obtained by our group showed that removal of 6 areas of the adipose tissue surrounding the thymus gland improved a complete remission rate, in comparison with removal of the thymus gland alone in patients with nonthymomatous MG (**Fig. 4**).[14] Our results of complete remission rate were consistent with results of Jaretzki[16] and Masaoka and colleagues.[17] Our second and even more important finding was that the chance of remission after maximally extended thymectomy

for nonthymomatous MG was still high in the presence of the ectopic foci in 3, 4, and even 5 areas of the adipose tissue of the lower neck/mediastinum[18] (**Fig. 5**), contrary to the results of Ashour,[19] and Ponseti and colleagues,[20] who reported that the chance for complete remission of MG was significantly lower in case of the presence of the ectopic foci.

There are several issues that make assessment of the role of thymectomy difficult.

It was confirmed in many cases that even incomplete thymectomy can lead to complete remission. It happens less often than in the case of complete extended thymectomy, nevertheless Papatestas and colleagues[3] reported approximately 24% of complete remissions after 5 years of follow-up after subtotal transcervical thymectomy. What is even more confusing, a complete remission also may occur in the course of purely medical treatment of MG, without any surgical procedure. All these taken together mean that probably there might be some critical mass of an immunologically active thymic tissue. If the treatment leads to reduction of this mass below the certain limit it causes that MG subsides. This might happen after successful thymectomy or immunosuppression. Are we able to assess this process? Currently, it is impossible, and we can only use some approximations, as was done by Jaretzki, who evaluated how radical were specific techniques of thymectomy and described a basic cervical thymectomy as removal of 40% to 50% of the whole thymic tissue up to 98% to 100%, with use of the transcervical-transsternal technique introduced by this author.[16] More radical procedures are connected with higher remission rates of MG after thymectomy. Currently, there is no specific imaging modality that could visualize ectopic foci of the thymic tissue. These foci can be discovered only during pathologic studies, and current knowledge on pathophysiology of MG is very

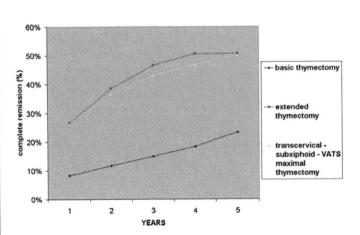

Fig. 4. Late results of basic transsternal, extended transsternal, and transcervical-subxiphoid-VATS maximal thymectomies; comparison of complete remission rates after 1, 2, 3, 4, and 5 years of follow-up. (*From* Zielinski M, Hauer L, Hauer J, et al. Comparison of complete remission rates after 5 year follow-up of three different techniques of thymectomy for myasthenia gravis. Eur J Cardiothorac Surg 2010;37:1141; with permission.)

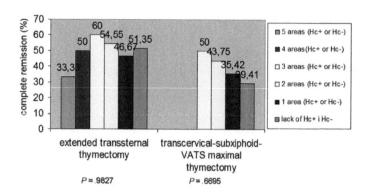

Fig. 5. Relationship between complete remission rates and the number of areas of the neck and the mediastinum in which ectopic thymic foci (Hc+ or Hc−) were discovered. Hc, Hassall corpuscles. (*From* Zieliński M. Definitions and standard indications of minimally-invasive techniques in thymic surgery. J Vis Surg 2017;3:99; with permission.)

incomplete. The role of the thymus is essential for development of the disease, but the whole process, including destruction of the acetylcholine receptors located on the postsynaptic membrane of the neuro-muscular junctions and subsequent regeneration of these receptors, is not known in every detail. It is very likely that even a complete removal of the thymus and the whole thymic tissue is not the sole factor leading to complete remission. The proponents of the minimally invasive techniques of thymectomy raised their advantages including a lesser burden of an operation, shorter hospitalization and recuperation, and, last but not least, a better cosmesis. For these reasons and especially due to avoidance of sternotomy, these approaches, especially the VATS technique, gained increasing popularity and challenged the role of transsternal thymectomy. Afterward, many articles supporting the efficacy of minimally invasive techniques of thymectomy were published worldwide. Finally, late results of surgical treatment of MG with minimally invasive techniques were claimed to be no different from those achieved with a transsternal thymectomy.[21,22] On the other hand, recent results from the US database suggested that hospital admissions for thymectomy in patients with nonthymomatous MG fell dramatically in this country after 2000.[12] One of the reasons might have been better immunotherapy; the other reasons were a reluctance of patients to undergo a major surgical thoracic procedure for the neurologic disease, lack of prospective randomized trials supporting the role of thymectomy for MG, and the last possible reason (never confirmed, but suspected) was an unsatisfactory effectiveness of minimally invasive techniques of thymectomy. Regarding the last objection, the explanation seems simple: good results reported by experts of minimally invasive thymectomy might be not repeated so successfully by average surgeons. Whatever was the reason

of decreasing number of thymectomies for nonthymomatous MG in the United States, and maybe in the other parts of the world, the results of a recently published prospective randomized trial comparing extended transsternal thymectomy, plus alternate-day prednisone with alternate-day prednisone alone, showing better results in the surgical arm, possibly might change positively the view of neurologists and myasthenic patients of the role of thymectomy.[12] The publication of the results of the prospective randomized trial comparing a medical treatment of MG with thymectomy provided evidence for a beneficial role of surgery performed in the extended transsternal technique. However, one must realize that the conclusions presented by Wolfe and colleagues[12] do not apply as a matter of course to the minimally invasive techniques of thymectomy.

The new question appears to be: does the superiority of transsternal thymectomy over medical treatment also valid for minimally invasive thymectomies?

A new prospective randomized trial comparing transsternal and minimally invasive thymectomies has been proposed to solve the problem.

It seems logical that to achieve equally good results, such a minimally invasive technique of thymectomy should be as extensive as the transsternal technique reported in the previously mentioned study. The surgical pattern of technique of transsternal extended thymectomy approved for the study of Wolfe and colleagues[12] was based on the technique described in detail by Jaretzki and Wolff,[7] which included a wide dissection of the mediastinal tissue of the lower part of the neck and the anterior mediastinum due to the presence of ectopic foci of the thymic tissue dispersed in there. One of the conclusions of Wolfe and colleagues[12] was that a randomized trial to compare transsternal and minimally invasive techniques of thymectomy was needed.

However, conduction of such a trial would be very difficult considering a variety of techniques of minimally invasive thymectomy. In other words, it would be difficult to compare a standardized extended transsternal technique with one of the variety of minimally invasive techniques of thymectomy. Analyzing this issue in detail, it would be difficult to explain why such a specific technique could be chosen, instead of many others and if it could represent all the other minimally invasive techniques of thymectomy? If the results of such technique were inferior than the results of the extended transsternal technique, would this mean that all minimally invasive techniques are inferior to the transsternal one?

Currently, there are no answers for these questions and, concluding, all uncertainties listed previously clearly show how much work is necessary to establish the role of thymectomy in the treatment of MG.

REFERENCES

1. Blalock A, Mason M, Morgan H, et al. Myasthenia gravis and tumors of the thymic region. Ann Surg 1939;110:544.
2. Crile G. Thymectomy through the neck. Surgery 1966;59:213.
3. Papatestas A, Genkins G, Kornfeld P, et al. Effects of thymectomy in myasthenia gravis. Ann Surg 1987; 206:79–88.
4. Masaoka A, Monden Y, Seike Y, et al. Reoperation after transcervical thymectomy for myasthenia gravis. Neurology 1982;32:83–5.
5. Henze A, Biberfeld P, Christiansen B, et al. Failing transcervical thymectomy in myasthenia gravis. Scand J Thorac Cardiovasc Surg 1984;18:235–8.
6. Masaoka A, Nagaoka Y, Kotake Y. Distribution of thymic tissue at the anterior mediastinum. Current procedures in thymectomy. J Thorac Cardiovasc Surg 1975;70:747–54.
7. Jaretzki A, Wolff M. "Maximal" thymectomy for myasthenia gravis. Surgical anatomy and operative technique. J Thorac Cardiovasc Surg 1988;96:711–6.
8. Cooper J, Al-Jalaihawa A, Pearson F, et al. An improved technique to facilitate transcervical thymectomy for myasthenia gravis. Ann Thorac Surg 1988;45:242–7.
9. Roviaro G, Rebuffat C, Varoli F, et al. Video thoracoscopic excision of mediastinal masses: indications and technique. Ann Thorac Surg 1994;58:1679–83.
10. Guyatt GH, Sackett DL, Cook DJ. Users' guides to the medical literature. II. How to use an article about therapy or prevention. B. What were the results and will they help me in caring for my patients? Evidence-Based Medicine Working Group. JAMA 1994;271:59–63.
11. Buckingham J, Howard F, Bernatz P, et al. The value of thymectomy in myasthenia gravis. A computer-assisted matched study. Ann Surg 1976;184:453–8.
12. Wolfe GI, Kaminski HJ, Aban IB, et al. Randomized trial of thymectomy in myasthenia gravis. N Engl J Med 2016;375:511–22.
13. Masaoka A, Monden Y. Comparison of the results of transsternal simple, transcervical simple, and extended thymectomy. Ann N Y Acad Sci 1981; 377:755–65.
14. Zielinski M, Hauer L, Hauer J, et al. Comparison of complete remission rates after 5 year follow-up of three different techniques of thymectomy for myasthenia gravis. Eur J Cardiothorac Surg 2010;37: 1137–43.
15. Mizia E, Klimek-Piotrowska W, Kużdżał J, et al. Residua of thymus in the mediastinum - clinical aspects - cadaveric study. Folia Med Cracov 2017; 57:23–8.
16. Jaretzki A. Thymectomy for myasthenia gravis: analysis of the controversies regarding technique and results. Neurology 1997;48(supl 5):S52–63.
17. Masaoka A, Yamakawa Y, Niwa H, et al. Extended thymectomy for myasthenia gravis patients: a 20-year review. Ann Thorac Surg 1996;62:853–9.
18. Zieliński M. Definitions and standard indications of minimally-invasive techniques in thymic surgery. J Vis Surg 2017;3:99.
19. Ashour M. Prevalence of ectopic thymic tissue in myasthenia gravis and its clinical significance. J Thorac Cardiovasc Surg 1995;109:632–5.
20. Ponseti JM, Gamez J, Vilallonga R, et al. Influence of ectopic thymic tissue on clinical outcome following extended thymectomy in generalized seropositive nonthymomatous myasthenia gravis. Eur J Cardiothorac Surg 2008;34:1062–7.
21. Mantegazza R, Confalonieri P, Antozzi C, et al. Video-assisted thoracoscopic extended thymectomy (VATET) in myasthenia gravis. Two year follow-up in 101 patients and comparison with the transsternal approach. Ann N Y Acad Sci 1998; 841:749–52.
22. Tomulescu V, Sgarbura O, Stanescu C, et al. Ten-year results of thoracoscopic unilateral extended thymectomy performed in nonthymomatous myasthenia gravis. Ann Surg 2011;254:761–5.

Surgical Techniques for Myasthenia Gravis
Video-Assisted Thoracic Surgery

Tommaso Claudio Mineo, MD[a,b,†],
Vincenzo Ambrogi, MD, PhD[b,c,d],*

KEYWORDS

• Thymectomy • VATS • Uniportal VATS • Myasthenia gravis • Thymoma

KEY POINTS

• Complete removal of thymus, perithymic tissue, and mediastinal fat is considered an effective treatment for improving the course of the myasthenia gravis.
• Thymectomy can be safely carried out by video-assisted thoracic surgery approach through 3 accesses as well as a unique surgical port.
• The procedures can be accomplished either bilaterally or unilaterally according to the surgeon's preference through the left or the right hemithorax.
• Whatever the video-assisted thoracic surgery approach results are equivalent in terms of operative trauma, perioperative and postoperative morbidity, hospital stay, patient's satisfaction, quality of life, and neurologic outcome as well.

INTRODUCTION

In 1941, describing the role of the thymus in myasthenia gravis (MG), Blalock wrote, "Complete removal of all thymic tissue offers the best chance of altering the course of the disease."[1] This was a relevant intuition of Blalock, supported over the years by other surgeons who can be considered pioneers in this field of thoracic surgery.[2–4]

Despite the lack of clear evidence and the absence of prospective randomized studies, thymectomy has increasingly gained credits as part of treatment for both thymomatous and nonthymomatous MG. Only in 2016, Wolfe and colleagues[5] published the first randomized prospective study regarding the role of thymectomy in nonthymomatous MG, which undeniably demonstrated the therapeutic benefit of surgery. At present, we have more certainties on the effectiveness of thymectomy in MG, although the exact mechanism determining the onset and remission of the disease is not yet fully understood. In addition, many other surgical issues, including patient selection, timing of surgery, appropriate approach, and impact of the procedure on the various myasthenic classes, remain undefined.

The presence of thymic elements outside the gland scattered in the mediastinum and in the neck,[6–9] evolved the concept of complete removal of all thymic tissue into Masaoka's "extended

Disclosure: The authors have nothing to disclose.
^a Department of Surgery and Experimental Medicine, Tor Vergata University, Via Montpellier 1, Rome 00133, Italy; ^b Myasthenia Gravis Multidisciplinary Program, Tor Vergata University, Viale Oxford 81, Rome 00133, Italy; ^c Department of Surgical Sciences, Tor Vergata University, Via Montpellier 1, Rome 00133, Italy; ^d Division of Thoracic Surgery, Tor Vergata University Policlinic, Viale Oxford 81, Rome 00133, Italy
[†] Deceased.
* Corresponding author. Division of Thoracic Surgery, Tor Vergata University Policlinic, Viale Oxford 81, 00133 Rome, Italy
E-mail address: ambrogi@med.uniroma2.it

Thorac Surg Clin 29 (2019) 165–175
https://doi.org/10.1016/j.thorsurg.2018.12.005

thymectomy"[10] and Jaretzki's "maximal thymectomy."[11]

For decades, transsternal and transcervical approaches had been the unique ways to accomplish thymectomy and their benefits and drawbacks are well-known.[12–14] Hitherto, the transsternal approach allows the most extended thymic tissue resection. The transcervical route can be considered the very first real minimally invasive approach.[15–17] However, the disadvantages of these approaches encouraged thoracic surgeons to find other solutions.

After the introduction of video-assisted thoracic surgery (VATS) in the early 1990s, this technique was rapidly applied to thymectomy. Since then, a variety of VATS procedures have been accomplished including left- or right-sided, unilateral or bilateral, triportal and uniportal, and ultimately subxiphoid approaches. These procedures boast shorter hospital stays, lower morbidity and mortality, decreased postoperative pain, and better cosmesis with equivalent efficacy when compared with open access procedures.

Herein, we describe the various VATS approaches to the thymus currently adopted in patients suffering from nonthymomatous and thymomatous MG.

ANATOMY FOR SURGEONS WHO PERFORM VIDEO-ASSISTED THORACIC SURGERY

A thorough knowledge of the anatomy of the thymus is of paramount importance to carry out safe thymectomy, avoiding incomplete operations or technical mishaps. This statement became vital in the current minimally invasive era, where the traditional direct vision is being replaced by a camera-mediated view in a restricted space, considerably limiting surgical maneuvers (**Figs. 1** and **2**). These conditions necessarily require a learning period after an adequate experience with sternotomy.

The thymus gland is approximately allocated in the midline of the anterosuperior mediastinum. In the adult, the gland appears as a lobulated structure including fat and glandular tissue. The gray ink color identifies the thymus in the diffuse yellow of mediastinal fat.

Despite wide variability, the thymus is usually formed by 2 longitudinal spindles of capsulated tissue fused in the middle, thus originating an asymmetric "H" with 4 projecting extremities named poles or horns, similar to a butterfly, as described by Sonett and colleagues.[18] In general, the lengths and sizes of the poles are different; the inferior right horn is larger than the left one, which is longer. The upper poles are thinner and reach

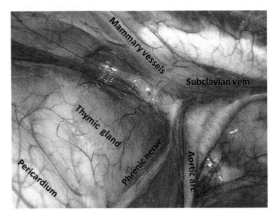

Fig. 1. Initial view from the left first port. The main anatomic landmarks are indicated.

the cervical area lying deep to the sternothyroid muscle in tight proximity to the recurrent laryngeal nerves.

The anatomic limits of the thymus are anteriorly the sternum; posteriorly the pericardium, the left innominate vein, and the trachea; laterally the mediastinal pleura up to the phrenic nerves; and cranially the cervical region up to the thyroid. Many anatomic variants are described, the most frequent being the innominate vein running anteriorly along the left superior horn.

The thymic arteries are tiny and inconstant; they originate from the internal mammary arteries and the inferior thyroid arteries. Venous drainage is much more evident; it takes place through 1 or 3 wide collectors that drain into inferior aspect of the innominate vein.

The thymus has an evident capsule that facilitates identification and smooth dissection from adjacent structures, but it may frequently form multilocated lobes in the perithymic tissue often separately encapsulated and distant.[18]

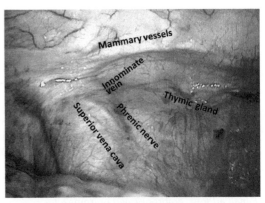

Fig. 2. Initial view from the right first port. The main anatomic landmarks are indicated.

Furthermore, unencapsulated thymic lobules and scattered microscopic foci may be variously found in the anterior mediastinal and pretracheal adipose tissue from the level of thyroid, above the diaphragm, along and beyond the phrenic nerves, and occasionally in the subcarenal fat.[7,9]

The goal of a successful thymectomy for MG is to remove as much thymic tissue as possible.[19] Thus, surgeons must know all the sites of thymic distribution within the mediastinum (**Figs. 3** and **4**). For better scientific standardization, we use a map specially created for this purpose.[20]

GENERAL ORGANIZATION

In 1986, at the Tor Vergata University of Rome was instituted the Thoracic Surgery Center. We soon created an MG Unit that became a Multidisciplinary Group, composed of surgeons, neurologists, anesthesiologists, intensive care physicians, physiotherapists, and nurses. We also involved external neurologists, physicians, and general practitioners, aiming to create a highly efficient structured network. This project entailed the evaluation of each myasthenic patient and the setting up of a computerized medical record to collect all demographic data, presenting symptoms, laboratory workups, imaging, informed consents, details of surgery, pathology, and follow-up data. We thus have the availability of a wide, up-to-date database that spans 3 decades.

ANESTHESIA

We have a dedicated anesthetic protocol for VATS thymectomy in myasthenic patients[20] with an anesthesiologist experienced in MG who personally evaluates each patient before the operation. All procedures are usually performed under

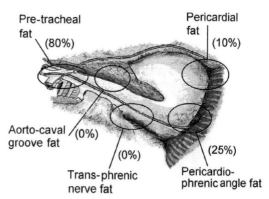

Fig. 4. Right view of the sites of ectopic thymic tissue. Within parentheses, the frequency rate for areas according to our experience.

general anesthesia with double lumen intubation confirmed by fiberoptic view and contralateral single-lung ventilation. More recently, we successfully used VATS thymectomy under nonintubated anesthesia and assisted ventilation through a laryngeal mask.

We monitor the patient intraoperatively with an electrocardiogram, noninvasive blood pressure, pulse oximetry, tidal capnometry, airways pressure, ventilator volume, train-of-four device for neuromuscular transmission and fraction of inspired oxygen. Intubation is performed without the use of muscle relaxant; the given inhaled anesthetics determine adequate relaxation. When required, a low dose of intermediate-acting nondepolarizing muscle relaxants can be supplemented. Depolarizing neuromuscular blocker agents should be avoided. Anticholinesterase drugs in the intraoperative and early postoperative period are administered through a nasogastric tube. A single stress dose of corticosteroid is usually inoculated before induction. Normocapnia is obtained by regulating ventilation frequency as well as volumes. As a consequence, early extubation and the resumption of spontaneous ventilation is achieved soon after surgery. After a short stay in the recovery unit, the anesthesiologist evaluates whether the patients can return to the ward or to the intensive care unit.

SURGERY

According the Myasthenia Gravis Foundation of America classification modified by Sonett and colleagues,[18] the classic VATS unilateral thymectomy is defined as T-2a, and the classic bilateral VATS without cervical incision as T-2c. These standardized definitions are useful in the evaluation of the outcomes. Herein, we describe the classic triportal left side, triportal right side, bilateral without

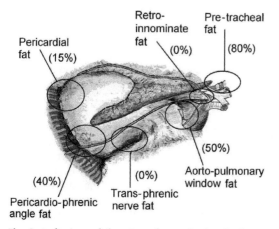

Fig. 3. Left view of the sites of ectopic thymic tissue. Within parentheses, the frequency rate for areas according to our experience.

cervical incision, and right or left uniportal approaches that we have experience with.

Patient Selection

Patients being considered for thymectomy must be medically optimized and educated to assume their anticholinergic medication at regular times. Preoperative treatment includes anticholinesterases, immunosuppressive agents, plasmapheresis, and intravenous immunotherapy. There are few contraindications to VATS thymectomy, such as morbid obesity, significant coagulopathy, prediction of thick bilateral pleural adhesions, and severe concomitant lung disease with an inability to tolerate single-lung ventilation. The ages recommended for thymectomy range from 10 and 60 years.[20] In general, better surgical results are achieved when symptoms have had a relatively recent onset and this is why we proposed thymectomy for those with class I MG.[21] All patients scheduled for an operation must be able to sustain a cycle of preoperative physiotherapy.[22]

Patient Position

Usually the patient lies in the semisupine decubitus with an elevated hemithorax of about 30° from the horizontal plane (**Fig. 5**), to allow for wider exposure of the anterior mediastinum. Usually, the ipsilateral arm is adducted and lowered below the trunk level to avoid interference with instruments. The patient is widely prepped and draped from the sternal notch to xiphoid to be ready for urgent sternotomy if it becomes necessary.

Surgeons and Equipment Position

The 2 operators stay on the same side of the chosen hemithorax, the operating surgeon in a

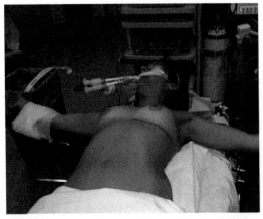

Fig. 5. Young myasthenic patient position for left uniportal video-assisted thoracic surgery thymectomy with the hemithorax raised 30°.

more cephalad position; the scrub nurse stands opposite to them. The anesthetic and videothoracoscopy units are positioned at the head of the patient. The suction unit, electrocautery, and additional energy devices are located to the side.

Instrument Armamentarium

Many instruments are common to open surgery, such as ring curved clamps, mounted pledget, right-angled clamp, as well as energy and either radiofrequency or ultrasound devices. Endoscopic instruments including endoclamps, endoscissors, endograspers, and endoclip appliers are useful. New dedicated instruments become necessary for uniportal access.

Classic Triportal Left-Side Video-Assisted Thoracic Surgery Thymectomy: T-2a

In 1993, we performed the first extended VATS thymectomy for nonthymomatous MG using a left-sided approach.[23] After we used this approach also for resection of early stage thymomas.[24] We have progressively modified the original technique to make thymectomy safer, faster, and more effective.[25]

Three trocars are inserted. The first 5- to 10-mm port is usually placed in the sixth intercostal space in the midaxillary line and a 30° videotelescope evaluates the collapse of the lung and the feasibility of the procedure. Two additional trocars are placed under vision: one located at the third intercostal space at the midaxillary line and the other at the sixth intercostal space anterior the axillary line. Blunt sponge may favor the lung collapse but carbon dioxide (CO_2) can be also insufflated from 8 to 12 mm Hg. In patients with a bulky adipose mediastinum predicted by chest magnetic resonance, we perform an adjuvant pneumomediastinum 24 hours preoperatively.[26]

We start by visualizing the left phrenic nerve along its entire way running over the lateral surface of the pericardium. Then, the aortopulmonary window, aortic arc, left internal mammary vessels, and innominate vein are progressively visualized. Pleural adhesions are released by using energy device. The mediastinal pleura is incised just anterior to the nerve and continues to the level of innominate vein and to inferior pole of the gland (**Fig. 6**). The left lower thymic horn is dissected free from the diaphragm, from the sternum and posteriorly from the pericardium along a clear and relatively avascular plan, until the right lung is discovered. Subsequently, dissection proceeds along the left internal mammary vein up to its confluence into the inferior border of the

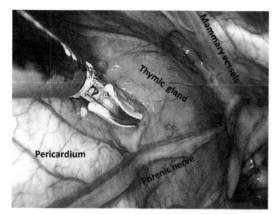

Fig. 6. Left-sided video-assisted thoracic surgery view. The left lower thymic horn is separated from the pericardium and dissected along the left phrenic nerve.

innominate vein, ensuring accurate sealing of the vessels from mammary artery. Injuries to nerves must be avoided because even transient unilateral palsy of the hemidiaphragm may be relevant in patients with MG. Now, we prefer complete clearance in the left pericardiophrenic angle from any residual adipose tissue.

At this stage, dissection continues over the pericardium until the right lower horn is exposed and freed from the pericardial surface (**Fig. 7**). In doing this, we recognize the contralateral mediastinal pleura by blunt technique, avoiding if possible entering into the pleural cavity. When necessary, the right pleural space can be opened and the lung intermittently ventilated, thus facilitating the identification of the right phrenic nerve. Hereby, the blunt dissection must include the right pericardiophrenic fat up to the right phrenic nerve, which is not always visible. At this step, care must be taken to identify vessels arising from the right internal mammary artery that can be divided safely by an energy device. The superior vena cava is then

exposed and all mediastinal tissue is carefully cleared off.

During surgery, we intermittently change the area of dissection thus avoiding insistent and unproductive action with risk of injuries. This technique also allows to refresh the view and reevaluate the progress in dissection, always checking the landmarks.

The mobilized inferior horns are lifted upward and laterally until the innominate vein confluence in superior vena cava is visualized. Total skeletonization of the vein is carefully done with a pledget exposing the thymic tributaries. In general, these are 2 or 3 small veins draining into the inferior border of the vein. They are safely divided by energy device (**Fig. 8**); larger veins need to be clipped. This step demands a supplementary caution to minimize the risk of bleeding, which can be compressed initially with a gauze on a clamp. If bleeding persists, the surgeon should consider a sternotomy or thoracotomy.

The 30° scope confirms the limit of right posterolateral previous dissection, also visualizing the right internal mammary vein that may by endoclipped to facilitate dissection of the upper horns. With the gland sufficiently mobilized, the superior horns are smoothly dissected in the cervical area that can be better visualized by flexion of the neck. If needed, an adjuvant cervical utility port may be used to widen the space and allow direct cervical dissection.

The left upper horn is dissected first in the extracapsular plan by a pledget dividing the small vessels from the neck with an energy device or endoclips (**Fig. 9**). An accessory horn lying under the innominate axis should be searched. Attention must be also paid to the recurrent laryngeal nerve, which runs in the tracheoesophageal groove, in proximity to the horn. Once freed the left upper horn, the right horn can be easily dissected and more distal vessels clipped or sealed (**Fig. 10**).

Fig. 7. Left-sided video-assisted thoracic surgery view. The right lower thymic horn is dissected from the pericardium surface until the contralateral pleura is visualized.

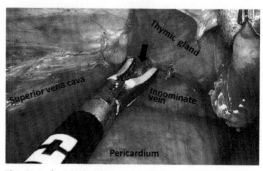

Fig. 8. Left-sided video-assisted thoracic surgery view. One thymic vein (*arrow*) is exposed by raising the freed thymus and sealed by energy device.

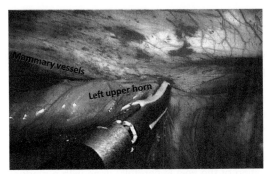

Fig. 9. Left-sided video-assisted thoracic surgery view. The left upper horn is isolated by pulling down the thymus.

The freed gland is placed in a retrieval bag and extracted from the most anterior and larger port or, in the case of a bulky thymus or thymoma, from an adjuvant supplementary subxiphoid incision. The specimen in both thymomatous and non-thymomatous thymectomy is always oriented and accurately inspected to confirm the integrity of the capsule. Any residual perithymic fat tissue is resected following our predefined map[20] and in particular from an aortopulmonary window, retro-innominate space, and where present beyond the left phrenic nerve.

Finally, hemostasis is carefully ensured by inspecting the dissected area and in particular around the vessels (**Fig. 11**). Any fluid collected in the pleural cavity is then removed. A chest tube may be placed in the thymic bed through the lower port.

Classic Triportal Right-Side Video-Assisted Thoracic Surgery Thymectomy: T-2a

To our knowledge, the right side triportal VATS was the first specific report of a minimally invasive

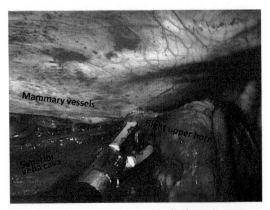

Fig. 10. Left-sided video-assisted thoracic surgery view. The right upper horn isolation by pulling the thymus downward and laterally.

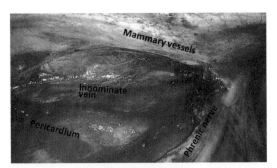

Fig. 11. Left-sided video-assisted thoracic surgery view. Final inspection of the thymic bed.

approach for thymectomy in patients with MG.[27] The advantage of the right side is the larger operative field, given the absence of the left ventricle, thus facilitating the vision of landmarks such as the right phrenic nerve, superior vena cava, innominate vein confluence, and right internal mammary vessels.

Port position is similar to the left-sided approach. Dissection starts by opening the mediastinal pleura from the right inferior horn proceeding cephalad along the phrenic nerve with blunt or energy dissection of the pericardial avascular plan until superior vena cava. We then dissect the right pericardiophrenic angle fat. The next step is to separate the gland from the sternum, following the right internal mammary vessels until the contralateral pleura is encountered, visualizing the inferior left horn, which is located deep in the left pericardiophrenic angle. Abundant fat tissue there present is extensively removed. The left lower horn is dissected free cephalad along the left phrenic nerve until the innominate vein, avoiding neural injuries. At this point, it is crucial to increase the visual field to be able to see past the ascending aorta. This goal can be conveniently achieved by laterally tilting the operative bed to raise the left hemithorax.

Gentle superior traction of the mobilized thymus allows easy dissection of the innominate axis until its confluence in the superior vena cava. Two or 3 sizable tributary veins draining the inferior aspect of innominate vein are carefully isolated and divided with an energy device. Larger veins may require vascular endoclips (**Fig. 12**). Accurate hemostasis of these vessels is mandatory to safely dissect the upper mediastinum and neck, where proper positioning of the 30° scope allows excellent visualization of the entire area. The right internal mammary vein sited at the brachiocephalic and superior vena caval junction may be endoclipped and divided to expose the superior horns.

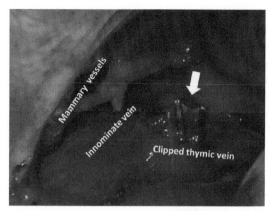

Fig. 12. Right-sided video-assisted thoracic surgery view. One large thymic vein is double clipped (*arrow*).

With a blunt dissection and delicate caudal traction of the freed gland, both superior horns can be mobilized from their fascial attachments and teased completely out of the neck (**Fig. 13**), having controlled small vessels emerging from the lower thyroid poles with an energy device. This step requires care to avoid injuries to the left recurrent laryngeal nerve. The patient's neck may be conveniently flexed by the anesthesiologist to facilitate dissection.

Finally, the entire gland can be removed as an en bloc specimen, including the mediastinal fatty tissue in an endobag via the most anterior port. Hemostasis is carefully ensured and the entire thymic bed inspected to ascertain the completeness of extended thymectomy according to our map. The aortopulmonary fat can be a site of ectopic immunogenic thymic tissue and therefore is carefully dissected free and separately retrieved.

Uniportal Video-Assisted Thoracic Surgery

Single-port VATS thymectomy may be reasonably considered as an evolution of the triportal VATS[28–30] and requires greater skill and synergism among the operator and the staff. This procedure can be approached from either side, according to surgeon preference.

The position of the surgeons is similar to that in the classic triportal VATS, but the operator might invert with the cameraman during the cervical steps. Dedicated instruments are mandatory, such as a long, double-hinged, narrow-shafted, and angulated tool for reaching the most cervical and contralateral areas avoiding wound crowding, knitting, torqueing, and interposition with a 30° thoracoscope. Recently, 180° and 3-dimensional view thoracoscopes have further simplified dissection.

The single incision is 3 or 4 cm long at the fourth or fifth intercostal space at the anterior–midaxillary line (**Fig. 14**). Incision longer than 6 cm can lose point of support for the instruments, whereas those smaller than 3 cm may cause interference. For better cosmesis, the incision should be lowered to be hidden under the bra or along the submammary fold. Larger incisions are required in obese patients, those with a thick chest wall, and those with a hypertrophic and neoplastic thymus as well.

The surgical wound should be always protected with a lubricated annular tissue retractor, which gently enlarges the space facilitating instrument insertion (**Fig. 15**). The thoracoscope should be kept at the most posterior end of the port. All surgical steps are similar to a triportal VATS; 1 instrument is used to hold the thymus and the other for dissection or suction.

In the right approach, the anterior mediastinum is first examined and major landmarks identified. The lower right horn, lower left horn, isthmus,

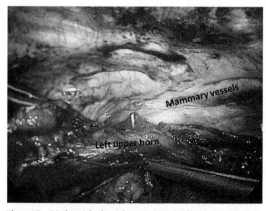

Fig. 13. Right-sided video-assisted thoracic surgery view. The left upper horn is isolated by an endodissector with the freed thymus gland pulled laterally.

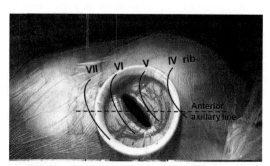

Fig. 14. Left uniportal video-assisted thoracic surgery thymectomy. The single incision is protected by a lubricated annular tissue retractor and sited at the fifth intercostal space to be hidden under the bra.

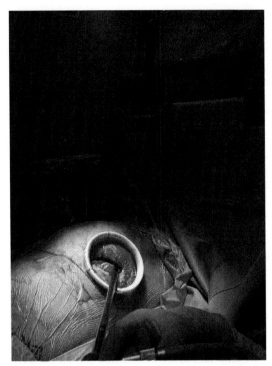

Fig. 15. Left uniportal video-assisted thoracic surgery thymectomy. Operative setting with camera sited in the most lateral end of the incision.

thymic veins, upper right horn, and upper left horn should be dissected sequentially by opportunely retracting the increasingly mobilized gland. The thymic vessels are divided as usual. This step demands supplementary caution to prevent intraoperative hemorrhages and conversion to open access. After the retrieval of en bloc thymus, we check hemostasis and remove extrathymic tissue following our map. A small drain is inserted in the anterior end of the wound to guarantee cosmesis.

For the left-sided approach, the setting is similar. Major landmarks are easily identified and surgical dissection is performed as described. Extra caution should be taken to identify the innominate vein, which is not immediately visible and is found at the junction between the internal mammary vessels and the left subclavian vein. By gentle dissection–traction, the entire innominate vein is exposed up to its confluence into the superior vena cava. Thymic veins are cauterized or endoclipped. Both superior horns are cautiously stripped down from the neck, avoiding injuries to the recurrent nerve. In the case of a large specimen, extraction may be accomplished through a subxiphoid incision. Afterward, the fat tissue in the right anterior mediastinum and right pericardiophrenic angle can be removed by opening the mediastinal pleura.

Bilateral Video-Assisted Thoracic Surgery Without Cervical Incision: T-2c

To achieve a more extended thymectomy some surgeons introduced a bilateral approach with and without an additional neck incision.[31–34] The first side to be approached changes according to the preference of the surgeon. The patient is usually placed in the supine position and widely prepped to be accessed on both sides. The table can be tilted from right to left or vice versa, with some degree of reverse Trendelenburg positioning. At the end of the first side step, a chest tube may be positioned according to the surgeon's preference.

Dissection follows the already described steps. Three ports are normally used for each side, although a uniportal approach on 1 side has been suggested.[35] The intraoperative variations are numerous: some authors prefers to deal with the thymic veins from the left approach first,[36] others start their dissection from the right side but divide the thymic veins from the left as final step,[37] and others dissect and divide the thymic veins from the right as an initial step.[33] There is not any full agreement regarding the benefit of an additional cervical (T-2b) because it is generally considered superfluous and less esthetically pleasing.[33]

Complications

Bleeding is undoubtedly the most notable complication. It can often be controlled by simple compression, but in case of persistence conversion to an open approach is mandatory. Sternotomy remains an essential skill for thoracic surgeons performing VATS thymectomy.

Completion Video-Assisted Thoracic Surgery Thymectomy

VATS completion thymectomies are performed in patients with refractory MG and suspected thymic residuals (**Fig. 16**). Unless originally performed via bilateral VATS, the contralateral side should be chosen to perform a completion thymectomy. In any case a different access from the previous one (ie, subxiphoid, transcervical) should be advisable. The operation broadly entails all the previously described steps, taking care to remove the predicted residual thymic tissue and to explore all the areas according to the map.

POSTOPERATIVE CARE

A sitting chest radiograph is taken 6 to 8 hours after surgery to rule out pneumothoraces or significant pleural collections, thus allowing chest drain removal. The neurology team is promptly involved

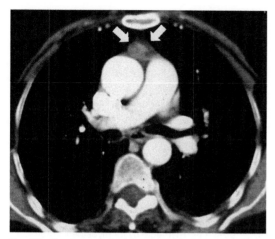

Fig. 16. Chest computed tomography scan showing a residual thymic area (*arrows*) in the aortocaval groove 2 years after left video-assisted thoracic surgery thymectomy.

after surgery to optimize myasthenic medications. Postoperative pain should be controlled adequately. A rehabilitation program is started immediately.[22] Patients are usually discharged within 3 days after surgery. The first follow-up visit is set within 3 to 4 weeks postoperatively.

COMMENT

When VATS broke onto the stage of thoracic surgery, it was soon evident that the thymus would have shortly become a notable target for minimally invasive procedures.[38] The relevant drawbacks of sternotomy and often limited radicality of the transcervical route significantly contributed to this process.

The main disadvantages of traditional access routes became instead prominent strengths of the minimally invasive surgery: less surgical trauma, decreased postoperative pain, a shorter hospital stay, faster return to normal activities, and an appreciably improved cosmetic results. Cosmesis was actually the main concern for young myasthenic girls and their neurologists, who were both often reluctant to consider surgery owing to disfiguring sternotomy scars.

VATS soon found favor with surgeons, allowing a very detailed vision of the surgical field that, although restricted, is wide enough for accomplishing accurate dissections thanks to the use of novel dedicated instruments. After an appropriate learning curve to get used to the lateral view, surgeons find VATS thymectomy increasingly safe and effective. VATS has proved to have several advantages over sternotomy, including decreased blood loss and operative time,[36] as well as a decreased incidence of postoperative

complications, namely, pulmonary infections.[37] Patients, neurologists, and general practitioners were also quick to appreciate these advantages.

Nowadays, VATS thymectomy procedures are various and controversies still exist regarding the most advantageous side of approach. However, the "laterality question" remains largely dependent on the surgeon's preference and experience, because an adequate extended thymectomy is achievable from either side.[23]

When comparing left- and right-sided approach to VATS thymectomy, similar operating times, postoperative complications, length of hospitalization, and rates of remission have been demonstrated.[39] No difference in operative complications were noted. The left side approach is preferred owing to the more prominent extent of mediastinal adipose tissue in the left side and the lesser probability of right phrenic nerve injury.

A right-sided approach was the preferred side from the beginning of VATS nonthymomatous thymectomy[27] and it is still prevalent in the literature.[36,37] This side entails a wider chest cavity, thus facilitating the surgical procedure. In addition, the superior vena cava serves as an immediate landmark, allowing for the rapid identification of the innominate vein and its tributaries.

Recently, uniportal VATS has gained in popularity among surgeons, proving to be safe and feasible.[30,40] Whatever side is chosen, this access route provides less chest trauma, improved cosmesis, and decreased costs.[28–30]

The unilaterality or bilaterality of the VATS procedure also remains another open issue. Because the fundamental goal of total thymectomy is to remove as much immunogenic thymic tissue as possible, some surgeons have successfully used a bilateral approach, advocating that a more complete thymectomy can be achieved.[32] Both sides of cardiophrenic fat tissue can be entirely excised, and the bilateral view might be especially useful in the event of a thymoma. The additional transcervical incision and neck dissection may favor a more extended removal of the immunogenic thymic tissue.[34] Unfortunately, a bilateral approach requires a longer operative time and causes much more pain than the unilateral one. In this regard, the novel subxiphoid approach[41] can allow for bilateral visualization and thymic clearance better than any unilateral approach, with less associated trauma and pain.

In our practice, we have tried all of these approaches and experienced the benefits and drawbacks. Our preference remains for the left VATS approach because it offers an excellent view of the entire thymic bed with better exposure of the aortopulmonary window, which is a frequent site of ectopic thymic tissue.[9,20] Ultimately, we undertook uniportal and subxiphoid VATS thymectomies as well. They require a considerable experience as well as a dedicated instrumentation, but can achieve better outcomes in terms of cosmesis and pain. Our vast experience with all VATS approaches makes us quite flexible to tailor minimally invasive thymectomies according to preoperative imaging findings or previous chest operations.

SUMMARY

At present, we are unable to clearly state which VATS access is the most advantageous in the prospective management of MG. Despite our preference for the left side, we would paradoxically recommend to a young surgeon to start with right triportal access. Indeed, this approach provides the wider space available in the right hemithorax and better visualization of the great vessels, thus decreasing the risk of vascular lesions. With increasing experience, we would advocate to undertake more complex routes, such as the single port from either side or the subxiphoid approach. On the basis of our long experience, we conclude that surgeons know all aspects of any approaches, but they should choose the route that suits them and their patient best.

REFERENCES

1. Blalock A, Harvey AM, Ford FF. The treatment of myasthenia gravis by removal of the thymus gland. JAMA 1941;117:1529–33.
2. Keynes G. The results of thymectomy in myasthenia gravis. Br Med J 1949;2:611–6.
3. Simpson JA. An evaluation of thymectomy in Myasthenia Gravis. Brain 1958;81:112.
4. Viets HR, Schwab RS. Thymectomy for Myasthenia Gravis. Springfield (IL): Charles C Thomas; 1960.
5. Wolfe GI, Kaminski AJ, Aban IB, et al. Randomized trial of thymectomy in myasthenia gravis. N Engl J Med 2016;375:511–22.
6. Masaoka A, Nagaoka Y, Kotake Y. Distribution of thymic tissue at the anterior mediastinum. Current procedures in thymectomy. J Thorac Cardiovasc Surg 1975;70:747–54.
7. Fukai I, Funato Y, Mizuno Y, et al. Distribution of thymic tissue in the mediastinal adipose tissue. J Thorac Cardiovasc Surg 1991;101:1099–102.
8. Ashour M. Prevalence of ectopic thymic tissue in myasthenia gravis and its clinical significance. J Thorac Cardiovasc Surg 1995;109:632–5.
9. Ambrogi V, Mineo TC. Active ectopic thymus predicts poor outcome after thymectomy in class III

myasthenia gravis. J Thorac Cardiovasc Surg 2012;143:601–6.
10. Masaoka A, Yamakawa Y, Niwa H, et al. Extended thymectomy for myasthenia gravis: a 20-year review. Ann Thorac Surg 1996;62:853–9.
11. Jaretzki A III, Wolff M. Maximal thymectomy for myasthenia gravis: surgical anatomy and operative technique. J Thorac Cardiovasc Surg 1988;96: 711–6.
12. Clagett OT, Eaton LM. Surgical treatment of myasthenia gravis. J Thorac Surg 1947;16:62–80.
13. Masaoka A, Monden Y. Comparison of the results of transternal simple, transcervical simple, and extended thymectomy. Ann N Y Acad Sci 1981; 377:755–65.
14. Jaretzki A III. Thymectomy for myasthenia gravis: an analysis of the controversies regarding technique and results. Neurology 1997;48:52–63.
15. Kirschner TA, Osserman KE, Kark AE. Studies in Myasthenia Gravis. Transcervical total thymectomy. JAMA 1969;209:906–10.
16. Papatestas AE, Genkins G, Kornfeld P, et al. Transcervical thymectomy in myasthenia gravis. Surg Gynecol Obstet 1975;140:535–40.
17. Mineo TC, Cirulli G, Rea S. La via transcervicale nella chirurgia del timo. Sett Ospedali 1978;20:59–63.
18. Sonett JR, Bromberger B, Jaretzki A III. Thymectomy for non thymomatous myasthenia gravis. In: Kaminski HJ, Kusner LL, editors. Myasthenia gravis and related disorders, current clinical neurology. New York: Humana Press; 2018. p. 199–219.
19. Jaretzki A III, Penn AS, Younger DS, et al. "Maximal" thymectomy for myasthenia gravis. Results. J Thorac Cardiovasc Surg 1988;95:747–57.
20. Mineo TC, Ambrogi V. Left VATS thymectomy. In: Mineo TC, editor. Novel challenges in Myasthenia Gravis. New York: Nova Science Publishers, Inc.; 2015. p. 415–49.
21. Mineo TC, Ambrogi V. Outcomes after thymectomy in class I myasthenia gravis. J Thorac Cardiovasc Surg 2013;145:1319–24.
22. Ambrogi V, Mineo TC. Benefits of comprehensive rehabilitation therapy in thymectomy for myasthenia gravis: a propensity score matching analysis. Am J Phys Med Rehabil 2017;96:77–83.
23. Mineo TC, Pompeo E, Ambrogi V. Video-assisted thoracoscopic thymectomy: from the right or from the left? J Thorac Cardiovasc Surg 1997;114:516–7.
24. Mineo TC, Sellitri F, Ambrogi V. Thymectomy for thymoma spanning three decades at Tor Vergata Thoracic Surgery Center. J Vis Surg 2018. https://doi.org/10.21037/jovs.2018.07.16.
25. Mineo TC, Sellitri F, Ambrogi V. Left-sided video-assisted thoracic surgery thymectomy. Video Assist Thorac Surg 2017;2:32.
26. Mineo TC, Pompeo E, Ambrogi V, et al. Adjuvant pneumomediastinum in thoracoscopic thymectomy

for myasthenia gravis. Ann Thorac Surg 1996;62: 1210–2.

27. Yim AP, Kay RL, Ho JK. Video-assisted thoracoscopic thymectomy for myasthenia gravis. Chest 1995;108:1440–3.

28. Ooi A, Qiang F. Uniportal video-assisted thoracoscopic surgery thymectomy (left approach). J Vis Surg 2016;2:12.

29. Ooi A, Sibayan M. Uniportal video-assisted thoracoscopic surgery thymectomy (right approach). J Vis Surg 2016;2:13.

30. Wu CF, Gonzalez-Rivas D. Uniportal video-assisted thoracoscopic thymectomy. Video Assist Thorac Surg 2017;2:25.

31. Lee CY, Kin DJ, Lee JG, et al. Bilateral video-assisted thoracoscopic thymectomy as a surgical extended thymectomy with more favorable early surgical outcomes for myasthenia gravis patients. Surg Endosc 2011;25:849–54.

32. Bromberger B, Sonett J. Bilateral VATS thymectomy in the treatment if myasthenia gravis. Video Assist Thorac Surg 2017;2:12.

33. Chang PC, Chou SH, Kao EL, et al. Bilateral video-assisted thoracoscopic thymectomy vs. extended transsternal thymectomy in myasthenia gravis: a prospective study. Eur Surg Res 2005;37:199–203.

34. Shigemura N, Shiono H, Inoue N, et al. Inclusion of the transcervical approach in video-assisted thoracoscopic extended thymectomy (VATET) for myasthenia gravis: a prospective trial. Surg Endosc 2006;20:1614–8.

35. Infante M, Benato C, Giovannetti R, et al. VATS thymectomy for early stage thymoma and myasthenia gravis: combined right-sided uniportal and left-sided three-portal approach. J Vis Surg 2017;3: 144.

36. Siwachat S, Tantraworasin A, Lapisatepun W, et al. Comparative clinical outcomes after thymectomy for myasthenia gravis: thoracoscopic versus transsternal approach. Asian J Surg 2018;41:77–85.

37. Gung Y, Zhang H, Li S, et al. Sternotomy versus video-assisted thoracoscopic surgery for thymectomy of myasthenia gravis patients: a meta-analysis. Asian J Endosc Surg 2016;9:285–94.

38. Magee MJ, Mack MJ. Surgical approaches to the thymus in patients with myasthenia gravis. Thorac Surg Clin 2009;19:83–9.

39. Tomulescu V, Sgarbura O, Stanescu C, et al. Ten-year results of thoracoscopic unilateral extended thymectomy performed in nonthymomatous myasthenia gravis. Ann Surg 2011;254:761–5.

40. Scarci M, Pardolesi A, Solli P. Uniportal video-assisted thoracic surgery thymectomy. Ann Cardiothorac Surg 2015;4:567–70.

41. Suda T. Subxiphoid uniportal video-assisted thoracoscopic surgery procedure. Thorac Surg Clin 2017;27:381–6.

Surgical Techniques for Myasthenia Gravis
Robotic-Assisted Thoracoscopic Surgery

Feng Li, MD[a], Mahmoud Ismail, MD[a], Aron Elsner, MD[a],
Deniz Uluk, MD[a], Gero Bauer, MD[a],
Andreas Meisel, MD, PhD[b], Jens-C. Rueckert, MD, PhD[a,*]

KEYWORDS

- Robotic-assisted thoracoscopic surgery • Thymectomy • Myasthenia gravis • Thymoma

KEY POINTS

- Robotic-assisted thoracoscopic surgery (RATS) creates an extended approach for thymectomy in terms of locating contralateral phrenic nerve and upper poles of the thymus.
- RATS thymectomy is indicated in all non-thymomatous myasthenia gravis (MG) patients and thymomatous MG patients with resectable thymoma, typically Masaoka-Koga I and II.
- Left-sided RATS thymectomy is superior for anatomic reasons: making the unreachable reachable.
- Left-sided RATS thymectomy is superior in the special care patients with MG: making the difficult easy.
- Left-sided three-trocar RATS thymectomy is the perfect combination of radical resection and minimal invasiveness among various approaches for thymectomy.

INTRODUCTION

Myasthenia gravis (MG) is a rare autoimmune disease that is characterized by fluctuating muscle weakness due to autoantibodies directing against the acetylcholine receptor (AChR) or other related functional molecules at the neuromuscular junction.[1] Thymectomy has become an alternative treatment of patients with MG since Blalock and colleagues[2] reported the first case treated with trans-sternal thymectomy in 1939. Thereafter, many approaches for thymectomy have been described, which can be mainly divided into 2 categories: open surgery (sternotomy, thoracotomy) and minimally invasive surgery (cervicotomy, video-assisted thoracoscopic surgery [VATS] and robot-assisted thoracoscopic surgery [RATS]).[2–6]

In 2016, the first randomized trial about thymectomy in patients with MG has demonstrated that extended trans-sternal thymectomy can improve the clinical outcomes and reduce the requirement of immunosuppressive medications in non-thymomatous MG patients seropositive for anti-AChR antibody.[7] Although extended trans-sternal thymectomy is still the golden standard of thymectomy, minimally invasive surgery for thymectomy has gained more and more popularity worldwide during the last decades.[8,9] Available data have demonstrated that RATS thymectomy is safe and feasible for patients with MG, as well as having a promising clinical outcome compared with other approaches.[10–12] However, long-term clinical outcome data are needed before considering RATS thymectomy a routine approach.

Disclosure: The authors have nothing to disclose.
a Department of Surgery, Competence Center of Thoracic Surgery, Charité University Hospital Berlin, Charité-platz 1, Berlin 10117, Germany; b Department of Neurology Berlin, Charité University Hospital Berlin, Charité-platz 1, Berlin 10115, Germany
* Corresponding author.
E-mail address: jens-c.rueckert@charite.de

The authors have been performing RATS thymectomy in patients with MG since 2003. Herein, we describe this approach in detail and discuss the technical tips, advantages, and disadvantages.

SURGICAL TECHNIQUES
Pre-operative Planning

The diagnosis of MG is confirmed through relevant symptoms and serum antibody assay.[1] Autoantibodies against AChR, muscle-specific tyrosine kinase, and low-density lipoprotein-related receptor 4 are specific and sensitive for the detection of MG.

In antibody-negative cases, electrophysiological tests (repetitive nerve stimulation or single-fiber electromyography) and/or the Tensilon test can secure the diagnosis.[13] Computed tomography is a routine imaging system used to assess the status of the thymus,[14] because about 10% of MG patients have a thymoma.[1] Also, previous studies have demonstrated that chemical shift magnetic resonance imaging can differentiate thymic hyperplasia from thymoma.[15,16]

With specialized treatment, symptomatic, immunosuppressive, and supportive therapy for MG have a good effect and the prognosis is generally good. All patients respond to acetylcholinesterase inhibition, and pyridostigmine is the first-line drug for the treatment of symptoms.[17,18] Most patients need immunosuppressive medications to reach full or nearly full physical function. Prednisone or prednisolone in combination with azathioprine is recommended as the first-line treatment.[17,18] Regarding supportive therapy and management, physical activity and systematic training should be recommended for patients with MG.[17,18] Besides, some drugs (such as muscle relaxants, penicillamine, and some antibiotics) should be avoided, if possible.

Indications

Thymectomy should be performed in MG patients with a thymoma to remove the tumor. RATS thymectomy is not routinely recommended in patients with thymoma, but may be considered if a complete resection with total thymectomy can be achieved, and if performed by experienced surgeons.[19–21] Previous studies have demonstrated that RATS thymectomy can be performed safely and effectively in both early-stage thymoma and large thymoma.[19–22] In non-thymomatous MG, thymectomy is performed as an option to potentially avoid or reduce the use of immunosuppressive medications, or if patients have failed to respond to those medications, or developed intolerable side effects from those medications.[17,18,23]

The authors have been performing RATS thymectomy in patients with MG since 2003 (**Fig. 1**). In MG patients without an anterior mediastinal lesion, left-sided approach for RATS thymectomy was the standard surgical approach for the authors. In MG patients with an anterior mediastinal lesion, the unilateral approach was chosen according to the location of the lesion.

Surgical Approach

In 2003, Ashton and colleagues[6] reported the first experience of RATS thymectomy in MG. Over

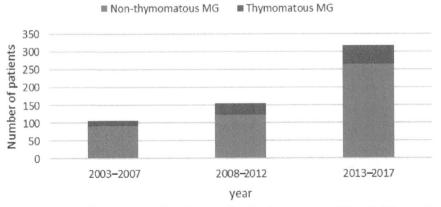

Fig. 1. Five hundred and eighty patients with MG, including 98 thymomatous MG and 472 non-thymomatous MG, underwent RATS thymectomy from 2003 to 2017 in Charité Universitaetsmedizin Berlin.

time, several approaches for RATS thymectomy have been reported, from unilateral, bilateral, to subxiphoid.[6,11,24,25] However, the discussion about whether to use a left- or right-sided approach for thymectomy has been ongoing for decades. Some surgeons prefer the left-sided approach because the left part of the thymic gland is usually larger and sometimes extending to or under the nerve. The aortopulmonary window, which is a frequent site of ectopic thymic tissue, is easier to address from the left side. The innominate vein runs mainly in the left anterosuperior mediastinum. Also, visualization of the contralateral phrenic nerve is easier from the left side.[26] On the other hand, surgeons who prefer the right-sided approach argue that identification of the superior vena cava, which allows easy identification of the left innominate vein favors the right side. Besides, the operative space is larger, which makes trocar placement easier and safer from the right side.[27] For unilateral RATS thymectomy, the pros and cons are similar to the unilateral VATS approach.

Since there has been controversy with regard to the completeness of resection achieved by minimally invasive approaches, the bilateral approach has been introduced to ensure radical resection.[24] Although a previous study has shown that unilateral VATS thymectomy offers equivalent clinical outcomes to that of the bilateral approach in patients with MG,[28] another study has demonstrated that bilateral RATS thymectomy is more likely to achieve a radical resection.[24] With regard to the so-called advantage of acquiring symmetric specimens, which is a reflection of radical resection in the study, we can technically harvest similar specimens using left-sided RATS thymectomy (**Fig. 2**).[24] Also, 2 drainage tubes, placed after the bilateral approach for thymectomy, can definitely cause more postoperative discomfort than one.

Subxiphoid RATS thymectomy has gained much attention and been increasingly applied in patients with MG during the last few years.[25,29] The advantages of this approach include minimizing the occurrence of intercostal neuropathy, sufficient visualization of the bilateral phrenic nerves and the cervical region, and, if necessary, rapid conversion to median sternotomy. For most patients, however, the subcostal instruments are not long enough to reach the upper poles of the thymus, which needs at least 1 robotic arm at the intercostal space to fix it.[25,29] Besides, because the cervical region is a frequent site of ectopic thymic tissue, concerns exist with regard to the long-term clinical outcome after subxiphoid RATS thymectomy.[30]

Of all the pros and cons, surgeons should always put the completeness of resection first, and consider the possible anatomic variations of every case regardless of the approach. However, with the advent of the da Vinci SP system, RATS thymectomy opens a new door to complete resection and minimal invasiveness (**Table 1**).

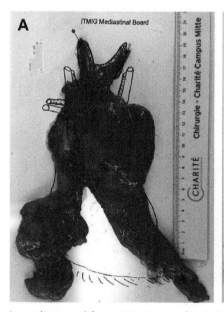
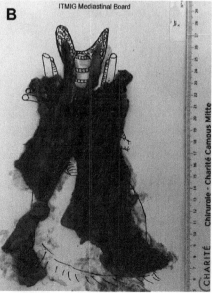

Fig. 2. Specimens harvested from MG patients after left-sided RATS thymectomy. (*A*) MG patient with a type B2, Masaoka-Koga I thymoma; (*B*) MG patient with thymic involution.

Table 1
Advantages of the da Vinci system

Items	Advantage
Visualization	Three-dimensional high-definition endoscope
Dexterity	Fully wristed and elbowed instruments
Precision and stability	Tremor filtration and fatigue avoidance
Minimal invasiveness	One incision with da Vinci SP
Workspace	Narrow access to anatomy anywhere
Nerve protection	ICG for nerve visualization

Preparation and Patient Positioning

Herein, the authors describe pre-operative preparation with regard to the left-sided approach. In brief, the skin was marked at the position of the trocar incisions in each case. Under general anesthesia, the patient was ventilated through a right-sided double lumen endotracheal tube. Subsequently, the patient was placed supine with the body moved to the left edge of the operating table, with the left arm placed parallel to the table and the right placed naturally along the body with the help of a vacuum beanbag

(**Fig. 3**A). Then the operative field was prepped, sterilized, and draped, exposing the chest from the left posterior axillary line to the right anterior axillary line to ensure there was enough area for conversion to sternotomy, if necessary (**Fig. 3**B). Thereafter, a 12-mm trocar, to which the 10-mm 30° angled camera was mounted, was inserted at the fourth intercostal space on the anterior axillary line, followed by insufflating carbon dioxide (CO_2) through it to a pressure of 8 mm Hg to achieve adequate visualization at the anterior mediastinum. Subsequently, the cranial special working trocar was inserted at the third intercostal space on the anterior axillary line with the help of the camera, followed by the caudal one at the fifth intercostal space between the midclavicular and the anterior axillary line (**Figs. 3**C, D). The da Vinci cart with robotic arms was then docked on the right side of the table, the central arm holding the camera, the cranial one connecting with an ultrasonic dissector, and the caudal one equipped with a precise bipolar forceps. The operator then sat at the console, which was prepared and positioned at some distance from the patient.

Surgical Procedure

For patients with an anterior mediastinal lesion, a meticulous inspection of the lesion is necessary before any dissection to evaluate the

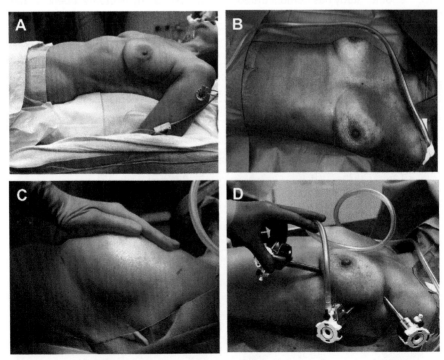

Fig. 3. Patient positioning with the help of a vacuum beanbag and trocar placement. (*A*) Patient was placed to the left edge of the operating table with the left arm placed parallel to the table. (*B*) The prepped, sterilized and draped operative field. (*C*) Skin marks for three trocars. (*D*) Port placements.

resectability of the lesion. Besides, thymectomy should be performed using a "no-touch" technique to minimize the risk of tumor seeding, which means the lesion should not be grasped or squeezed during the operation.[31] Furthermore, the surgical margins should be analyzed by the pathologist to assess the completeness of the resection.[31]

In brief, resection in this procedure starts in the middle of the pericardium and moves cranially along the nerve (**Figs. 4**A–C). Because the thymic gland can cross the border of the phrenic nerve in some cases, and that this anatomic variation can be found exclusively at the left side, surgeons should ensure protection of the phrenic nerve during the dissection until it is completely isolated from the mediastinal tissue.

Subsequently, the tissue in the aortopulmonary window is mobilized and the dissection proceeds upward to the lower cervical region until the cervical pleura is opened at the entrance to the left innominate vein. The pleura incision is extended to the mediastinal retrosternal line. Then the incision proceeds to the right side until the subxiphoid pleural fold is reached and the right lung is visible (**Figs. 4**D, E). Extra care should be given to avoid opening the right pleural cavity too early, otherwise the option of enlarging the operation field by CO_2 will be lost.

The next step is to manage the upper poles: bringing them down by grasping and retracting

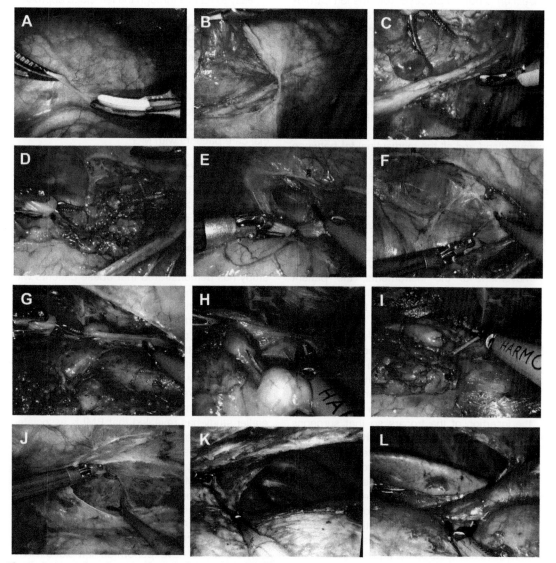

Fig. 4. Presentative pictures of surgical procedure. (*A-C*) Resection starts in the middle of the pericardium and moves cranially along the nerve. (*D-F*) The incision proceeds to the right side until the right lung is visible, but the right pleural cavity is still closed. (*G-I*) Management of the upper poles and thymic veins. (*J-L*) Open the right pleural cavity and the cardiophrenic tissue is dissected completely with clear visualization of the right phrenic nerve.

carefully before dissecting them bluntly from the inferior portion of the thyroid gland. Two grasping instruments are essential here. After identification of the left innominate vein by handling the left upper pole, the dissection continues meticulously along the innominate vein to identify and dissect the thymic veins (**Figs. 4**F–H). Utmost attention should be paid to the atypically located thymic veins. The dissection is made using a harmonic scalpel; clips are no longer required.

After mobilizing all of the median retrosternal tissue, the right main thymic lobe can be visualized in the aortocaval groove. Thereafter, the tissue in the left cardiophrenic angle is completely dissected and moved upward. The last strategic step of the dissection is now to proceed from the left cardiophrenic angle to the subxiphoid area, and subsequently to the right cardiophrenic area, where the right pleura is then opened and the cardiophrenic tissue can be dissected completely with clear visualization (**Figs. 4**I–K).

Since this approach provides a clear operative visualization of the contralateral phrenic nerve, operators are able to manage the right-sided dissection maximally and safely. After resecting the thymus gland and all the mediastinal fat between the phrenic nerves from diaphragm to lower cervical area radically, the whole specimen is then placed in an endobag for removal through the 12-mm port incision.

Technical Tips

1. *Patient positioning*. To get enough space for movement of the instruments, the patient should be placed supine with the body moved to the left edge of the operating table, lowering the left arm to be parallel to the table and placing the right one naturally along the body.
2. *Trocar placement*. Some surgeons prefer the right-sided approach because of concerns about lacerating the pericardium, or even the heart, while inserting the trocars through the left side.[32] Use of a shear can help to guide the insertion of the trocars so that surgeons can always control the depth of the trocar insertion easily. After placement of the 12-mm camera trocar, insufflation with CO_2 to a pressure of 8 mm Hg is carried out to enlarge the retrosternal space for the insertion of the other trocars under the view of the camera. For the inexperienced, using a spatula to push the heart aside or to moderately lift the camera is also effective to acquire adequate space and ensure the safe placement of the trocars.
3. *Thymic upper pole resection*. The upper poles are freed from the innominate vein and upper

mediastinum; bringing them down by retraction before resection is an effective way to manage the upper poles, which is essential for a radical thymectomy.
4. *Thymic vein management*. Although anatomic variations occur in some cases, there are usually 2 to 3 thymic veins running about 2 cm before draining into the left innominate vein.[33] Therefore, special attention should be paid to identify the left innominate vein to avoid the injury of the thymic veins and the innominate vein. The left innominate/superior vena cava angle is a common site for a thymic vein. Also, common anatomic variations occur at the upper left horn and run behind the innominate vein, which is easy to handle through the left-sided approach.

EXPERIENCE OF ROBOTIC-ASSISTED THORACOSCOPIC SURGERY THYMECTOMY IN SPECIAL CARE PATIENTS WITH MYASTHENIA GRAVIS

As well as the advantages from the da Vinci system (see **Table 1**), the left-sided approach for RATS thymectomy is also safe and feasible in special care patients with MG.

Obese Patients with Myasthenia Gravis

Obesity adds special risks for thoracic surgery procedures because of obesity-related comorbidities and physical body habitus.[34] A previous study has shown that higher body mass index (BMI) (>28 kg/m^2) is independently associated with postoperative myasthenic crisis.[35] Also, another study has demonstrated that obese patients with MG have a higher risk of postoperative complications after trans-sternal thymectomy.[36] On the other hand, performing thymectomy in obese patients with MG poses challenges from a technical standpoint. Extra-long trocars need to be introduced, and extra care must be taken to avoid any injury of the vital structures during their placement. Also, increased body mass may limit visualization and range of instrument movement. An earlier study has revealed that BMI is associated with longer operation time for VATS thymectomy.[37] Thus, special considerations should be taken when planning a thymectomy on obese patients with MG. Because the da Vinci system can provide a better visualization, enhanced dexterity, and precision for thymectomy, the authors consider that RATS thymectomy can be conducted in obese patients in an easy and safe manner.

The authors have performed left-sided RATS thymectomy in 69 MG patients with a high BMI (≥30 kg/m^2) from 2003 to 2017. Perioperative complications occurred in 6 (8.7%) patients (**Table 2**).

Table 2
Complications resulting from RATS thymectomy in 69 MG patients with a high BMI ($\geq$30 kg/m^2)

Gender	Age at Onset (yr)	BMI Pre-ThX (kg/m^2)	Delay of ThX (mo)	MGFA Class	Thymic Pathology	Postoperative Complication	Concomitant Disease Pre-ThX[a]
Male	55	32.3	12	I	Involution	Chylothorax	Hypertension
Male	46	31	19	IIa	Involution	Hypokalemia	No
Male	57	31.1	84	I	Involution	Arrhythmia	CHD, DM, hypertension, arrhythmia
Male	72	34	3	I	Thymoma	Pleural effusion	CHD, DM, hypertension, arrhythmia
Male	66	30.1	2	IIb	Involution	Atrial fibrillation	CHD, DM, hypertension, arrhythmia
Female	62	51.1	4	I	Thymoma	Respiratory failure	Hypertension, DM

Abbreviations: CHD, coronary heart disease; DM, diabetes mellitus; MG, myasthenia gravis; ThX, thymectomy.
[a] Concomitant disease here includes hypertension, DM, CHD, and arrhythmia.

No perioperative mortality was observed in this series. Therefore, the authors recommend left-sided RATS thymectomy as a superior approach in this situation, in which thymectomy can be conducted safely and easily. However, extra attention should be paid to pre-operative assessment, especially history and examinations of cardiac and pulmonary comorbidities. Also, utmost care should be given to reduce or avoid postoperative complications that require adequate pain control, so that mobilization and vigorous coughing can begin early after thymectomy.

Children with Prepubertal Myasthenia Gravis Onset

Thymectomy is also a treatment option in children with prepubertal MG onset (age < 12 years).[17,18,23] A pediatric neurologic perspective is required before planning a thymectomy in a pediatric population, because MG patients with prepubertal onset have different clinical features and responses to therapy. Although the role of thymectomy in children is controversial due to the immunologic function of thymus, previous studies have not found any negative effect of thymectomy on acquired immune function.[38,39] Corticosteroids, however, do have a negative effect on growth and bone mineralization in juvenile MG.[40] Up to now, several approaches for thymectomy have been described in children, and 1 study has also demonstrated that VATS thymectomy might result in a lower perioperative morbidity compared with the trans-sternal approach.[41,42] RATS thymectomy has similar benefits as VATS, but also offers a three-dimensional visualization and has the highest-dexterity and articulating arms that provide easier access to the contralateral phrenic

nerve and upper poles of the thymus. Because children have a relatively large thymus in a small chest cavity, and that RATS thymectomy is perfect to work in a confined space, the authors think that RATS thymectomy can be safely and easily performed in children with MG.

Seventeen MG patients with prepubertal onset (1–11 years old) underwent left-sided RATS thymectomy from 2003 to 2017. Perioperative morbidity occurred in 1 (5.9%) patient: chylothorax, similar to that previously reported after VATS thymectomy.[41] The results indicated that RATS thymectomy could be performed with a low perioperative morbidity in children as young as 1 year old. Apart from the confined operative space, the relatively large thymus is located anatomically close to the surrounding vital structures in the anterior mediastinum in children. Thus, precise dissection is required when performing a thymectomy in these cases. The authors recommend RATS thymectomy in children with MG in whom thymectomy can be performed with a complete and precise resection.

Re-thymectomy in Patients with Myasthenia Gravis

In some MG patients, myasthenic symptoms subside temporarily or even remain the same after thymectomy. Treatment options are limited in these patients because of the difficult-to-control symptoms. These patients are usually considered as refractory MG. Residual thymic tissue is present in most of these refractory MG patients after thymectomy.[43–45] Previous studies have demonstrated that this is likely due to an incomplete resection or development of ectopic thymic tissue.[45] Repeat thymectomy is a treatment option in these

Table 3
Clinical parameters of 5 re-thymectomy patients with MG

Case No.	Gender	Age at Onset (yr)	First ThX Delay (mo)	First ThX Approach	Interval Between Operations (mo)	Re-ThX Approach	Tissue Weight After Re-ThX (g)	Pathology of Thymus After Re-ThX
1	Man	14	48	Sternotomy	144	RATS	31	Follicular hyperplasia
2	Woman	18	84	VATS	84	RATS	23	Involution
3	Woman	42	4	Sternotofmy	24	RATS	14	Normal thymic tissue
4	Man	52	84	VATS	171	RATS	15	B2 thymoma
5	Woman	8	6	Cervicotomy	132	RATS	26	No thymic tissue

Abbreviations: RATS, robot-assisted thoracoscopic surgery approach for thymectomy; ThX, thymectomy; VATS, video-assisted thoracoscopic surgery approach for thymectomy.

patients. Re-operation has been mostly carried out through aggressive trans-sternal approaches in some small series.[46] However, these invasive approaches may result in high postoperative morbidity, and 1 study has reported that injury of the innominate vein at re-sternotomy occurred in 3 (14.3%) patients.[46,47] Therefore, VATS thymectomy has been recently investigated in the belief that it may achieve a complete resection in a less-aggressive way.[45] However, 2 patients had myasthenic crisis requiring ventilation in the postoperative period after VATS re-thymectomy.[45] On the other hand, although the recurrence of thymoma is rare after thymectomy, available data have shown that re-operation is feasible, with acceptable morbidity and low mortality in selected patients with locally recurrent thymoma.[48] Also, morbidity and mortality during re-thymectomy are more likely to occur in patients with MG,[48] with mobilization of the adhesions at re-thymectomy sometimes adding difficulty for the procedure. As the latest advance in minimally invasive surgery, RATS thymectomy has been reported to be a less-aggressive approach with regard to surgical trauma with a complete resection.[11,12,29] With this in mind, we have adopted this approach to re-operate on refractory MG patients or MG patients with recurrent thymoma.

The authors have performed RATS re-thymectomy in 5 MG patients with or without thymoma from 2003 to 2017 (**Table 3**). Neither perioperative morbidity (including MG crises) nor conversion to open surgery was observed in this series. Case 5 underwent thymectomy 3 times through cervicotomy, sternotomy, and RATS approaches at 6, 11, and 138 months after MG onset, respectively. Specimens from the first 2 thymectomies showed follicular hyperplasia with no evidence of a thymoma. Although the case series was quite small, it shed light on the safety and feasibility of RATS re-thymectomy in refractory MG patients and MG patients with recurrent thymoma.

Left-sided RATS thymectomy is superior in patients with MG because it makes unreachable areas reachable and difficult cases easy, which offers surgeons the best chance for a complete resection and patients the best chance for remission.

DISADVANTAGES OF ROBOTIC-ASSISTED THORACOSCOPIC SURGERY THYMECTOMY

Compared with non-RATS thymectomy, increased docking time and high cost are obviously the common disadvantages of all approaches using RATS thymectomy. Furthermore, if there is any emergency, such as major bleeding, that requires open conversion, the undocking of the robotic system and the sterilization of the operator consume much valuable time, possibly resulting in the emergency being more difficult to manage.

SUMMARY

Extended thymectomy is effective in improving clinical outcomes in patients with MG. In the era of minimally invasive surgery, most MG patients undergo thymectomy through VATS or RATS approaches. RATS thymectomy, especially with the da Vinci SP system, is the perfect combination of radical resection and minimal invasiveness among various approaches for thymectomy. Up to now, the authors have recommended left-sided three-trocar RATS thymectomy as a superior approach in patients with MG. However, comparative studies about long-term clinical outcomes of MG patients after different RATS approaches for thymectomy are still missing. Future studies should focus on comparison of different surgical approaches with long-term follow-up.

REFERENCES

1. Gilhus NE. Myasthenia gravis. N Engl J Med 2016; 375(26):2570–81.
2. Blalock A, Mason MF, Morgan HJ, et al. Myasthenia gravis and tumors of the thymic region: report of a case in which the tumor was removed. Ann Surg 1939;110(4):544–61.
3. Kark AE, Kirschner PA. Total thymectomy by the transcervical approach. Br J Surg 1971;58(5):321–6.
4. Mineo TC, Pompeo E, Ambrogi V, et al. Adjuvant pneumomediastinum in thoracoscopic thymectomy for myasthenia gravis. Ann Thorac Surg 1996; 62(4):1210–2.
5. Zielinski M. Technique of transcervical-subxiphoid-vats "maximal" thymectomy in treatment of myasthenia gravis. Przegl Lek 2000;57(Suppl 5):64–5.
6. Ashton RC Jr, McGinnis KM, Connery CP, et al. Totally endoscopic robotic thymectomy for myasthenia gravis. Ann Thorac Surg 2003;75(2):569–71.
7. Wolfe GI, Kaminski HJ, Aban IB, et al. Randomized trial of thymectomy in myasthenia gravis. N Engl J Med 2016;375(6):511–22.
8. Jaretzki A 3rd. Thymectomy for myasthenia gravis: analysis of controversies–patient management. Neurologist 2003;9(2):77–92.
9. Marulli G, Schiavon M, Perissinotto E, et al. Surgical and neurologic outcomes after robotic thymectomy in 100 consecutive patients with myasthenia gravis. J Thorac Cardiovasc Surg 2013;145(3):730–5.
10. Renaud S, Santelmo N, Renaud M, et al. Robotic-assisted thymectomy with da Vinci II versus sternotomy in the surgical treatment of non-thymomatous myasthenia gravis: early results. Rev Neurol (Paris) 2013;169(1):30–6.
11. Ruckert JC, Swierzy M, Ismail M. Comparison of robotic and nonrobotic thoracoscopic thymectomy: a cohort study. J Thorac Cardiovasc Surg 2011;141(3):673–7.
12. Freeman RK, Ascioti AJ, Van Woerkom JM, et al. Long-term follow-up after robotic thymectomy for nonthymomatous myasthenia gravis. Ann Thorac Surg 2011;92(3):1018–22.
13. Chiou-Tan FY, Gilchrist JM. Repetitive nerve stimulation and single-fiber electromyography in the evaluation of patients with suspected myasthenia gravis or Lambert-Eaton myasthenic syndrome: review of recent literature. Muscle Nerve 2015;52(3):455–62.
14. Ottlakan A, Borda B, Morvay Z, et al. The effect of diagnostic imaging on surgical treatment planning in diseases of the thymus. Contrast Media Mol Imaging 2017;2017:9307292.
15. Popa GA, Preda EM, Scheau C, et al. Updates in MRI characterization of the thymus in myasthenic patients. J Med Life 2012;5(2):206–10.
16. Priola AM, Priola SM, Gned D, et al. Comparison of CT and chemical-shift MRI for differentiating thymoma from non-thymomatous conditions in myasthenia gravis: value of qualitative and quantitative assessment. Clin Radiol 2016;71(3):e157–69.
17. Sanders DB, Wolfe GI, Benatar M, et al. International consensus guidance for management of myasthenia gravis: executive summary. Neurology 2016;87(4): 419–25.
18. Gilhus NE, Verschuuren JJ. Myasthenia gravis: subgroup classification and therapeutic strategies. Lancet Neurol 2015;14(10):1023–36.
19. Liu TJ, Lin MW, Hsieh MS, et al. Video-assisted thoracoscopic surgical thymectomy to treat early thymoma: a comparison with the conventional transsternal approach. Ann Surg Oncol 2014;21(1): 322–8.
20. Pennathur A, Qureshi I, Schuchert MJ, et al. Comparison of surgical techniques for early-stage thymoma: feasibility of minimally invasive thymectomy and comparison with open resection. J Thorac Cardiovasc Surg 2011;141(3):694–701.
21. Ye B, Tantai JC, Ge XX, et al. Surgical techniques for early-stage thymoma: video-assisted thoracoscopic thymectomy versus transsternal thymectomy. J Thorac Cardiovasc Surg 2014;147(5):1599–603.
22. Kneuertz PJ, Kamel MK, Stiles BM, et al. Robotic thymectomy is feasible for large thymomas: a propensity-matched comparison. Ann Thorac Surg 2017;104(5):1673–8.
23. Sanders DB, Wolfe GI, Narayanaswami P, MGFA Task Force on MG Treatment Guidance. Developing treatment guidelines for myasthenia gravis. Ann N Y Acad Sci 2018;1412(1):95–101.
24. Kawaguchi K, Fukui T, Nakamura S, et al. A bilateral approach to extended thymectomy using the da Vinci Surgical System for patients with myasthenia gravis. Surg Today 2018;48(2):195–9.
25. Suda T, Tochii D, Tochii S, et al. Trans-subxiphoid robotic thymectomy. Interact Cardiovasc Thorac Surg 2015;20(5):669–71.
26. Mineo TC, Pompeo E, Ambrogi V. Video-assisted thoracoscopic thymectomy: from the right or from the left? J Thorac Cardiovasc Surg 1997;114(3):516–7.
27. Cerfolio RJ, Bryant AS, Minnich DJ. Starting a robotic program in general thoracic surgery: why, how, and lessons learned. Ann Thorac Surg 2011; 91(6):1729–36 [discussion: 36–7].
28. Liu Z, Yang J, Lin L, et al. Unilateral video-assisted thoracoscopic extended thymectomy offers long-term outcomes equivalent to that of the bilateral approach in the treatment of non-thymomatous myasthenia gravis. Interact Cardiovasc Thorac Surg 2015;21(5):610–5.
29. Zhang H, Chen L, Zheng Y, et al. Robot-assisted thymectomy via subxiphoid approach: technical details and early outcomes. J Thorac Dis 2018;10(3): 1677–82.
30. Ambrogi V, Mineo TC. Active ectopic thymus predicts poor outcome after thymectomy in class III

myasthenia gravis. J Thorac Cardiovasc Surg 2012; 143(3):601–6.

31. Toker A, Sonett J, Zielinski M, et al. Standard terms, definitions, and policies for minimally invasive resection of thymoma. J Thorac Oncol 2011;6(7 Suppl 3): S1739–42.

32. Marulli G, Rea F, Melfi F, et al. Robot-aided thoracoscopic thymectomy for early-stage thymoma: a multicenter European study. J Thorac Cardiovasc Surg 2012;144(5):1125–30.

33. Yune HY, Klatte EC. Thymic venography. Radiology 1970;96(3):521–6.

34. Liou DZ, Berry MF. Thoracic surgery considerations in obese patients. Thorac Surg Clin 2018;28(1): 27–41.

35. Leuzzi G, Meacci E, Cusumano G, et al. Thymectomy in myasthenia gravis: proposal for a predictive score of postoperative myasthenic crisis. Eur J Cardiothorac Surg 2014;45(4):e76–88 [discussion: e88].

36. Liu XD, Shao MR, Sun L, et al. Influence of body mass index on postoperative complications after thymectomy in myasthenia gravis patients. Oncotarget 2017;8(55):94944–50.

37. Toker A, Tanju S, Ziyade S, et al. Learning curve in videothoracoscopic thymectomy: how many operations and in which situations? Eur J Cardiothorac Surg 2008;34(1):155–8.

38. Ionita CM, Acsadi G. Management of juvenile myasthenia gravis. Pediatr Neurol 2013;48(2):95–104.

39. Sauce D, Larsen M, Fastenackels S, et al. Evidence of premature immune aging in patients thymectomized during early childhood. J Clin Invest 2009; 119(10):3070–8.

40. Wang H, Su Z, Luo C, et al. The effect of steroid treatment and thymectomy on bone age and height development in juvenile myasthenia gravis. Neurol Sci 2013;34(12):2173–80.

41. Goldstein SD, Culbertson NT, Garrett D, et al. Thymectomy for myasthenia gravis in children: a comparison of open and thoracoscopic approaches. J Pediatr Surg 2015;50(1):92–7.

42. Hartwich J, Tyagi S, Margaron F, et al. Robot-assisted thoracoscopic thymectomy for treating myasthenia gravis in children. J Laparoendosc Adv Surg Tech A 2012;22(9):925–9.

43. Husain F, Ryan NJ, Hogan GR, et al. Occurrence of invasive thymoma after thymectomy for myasthenia gravis: report of a case. Neurology 1990;40(1): 170–1.

44. Rosenberg M, Jauregui WO, Herrera MR, et al. Recurrence of thymic hyperplasia after transsternal thymectomy in myasthenia gravis. Chest 1986;89(6):888–9.

45. Mineo TC, Pompeo E, Ambrogi V, et al. Video-assisted completion thymectomy in refractory myasthenia gravis. J Thorac Cardiovasc Surg 1998;115(1): 252–4.

46. Zielinski M, Kuzdzal J, Staniec B, et al. Extended rethymectomy in the treatment of refractory myasthenia gravis: original video-assisted technique of resternotomy and results of the treatment in 21 patients. Interact Cardiovasc Thorac Surg 2004;3(2): 376–80.

47. Bulkley GB, Bass KN, Stephenson GR, et al. Extended cervicomediastinal thymectomy in the integrated management of myasthenia gravis. Ann Surg 1997;226(3):324–34 [discussion: 34–5].

48. Dai J, Song N, Yang Y, et al. Is it valuable and safe to perform reoperation for recurrent thymoma? Interact Cardiovasc Thorac Surg 2015;21(4): 526–31.

Uniportal Video-Assisted Transcervical Thymectomy

Philippe H. Lemaître, MD[a], Shaf Keshavjee, MD[b],*

KEYWORDS

- Myasthenia gravis • Thymectomy • Transcervical • VATS

KEY POINTS

- Surgery has proven superiority over medical management for patients with nonthymomatous myasthenia gravis.
- The key is complete resection of the gland, which can be achieved with various techniques.
- The uniportal video-assisted transcervical technique allows minimally invasive surgery with a low complication rate, a good cosmetic result, and a short length of recovery.

Myasthenia gravis (MG) is an autoimmune disease in which antibodies (Abs) bind to acetylcholine receptors (AChRs) or to functionally related molecules in the postsynaptic membrane at the neuromuscular junction, leading to impaired neuromuscular transmission and muscle weakness.[1] Eighty to ninety percent of patients with MG have AChR-Abs. The other two principal targets are muscle-specific tyrosine kinase (MuSK), a transmembrane component of the postsynaptic neuromuscular junction, and lipoprotein-related protein 4 (LRP4), part of the MuSK complex.[1]

Fatigable weakness is the clinical hallmark of MG, with a predilection for the ocular and bulbar muscles, although generalized proximal muscle weakness is also common. The disorder is diagnosed by the clinical presentation, abnormal single-fiber electromyography, repetitive nerve-stimulation tests, and elevated AChR and/or anti-MuSK antibodies. Abnormalities of the thymus gland are commonly found in these patients. Lymphoid thymic hyperplasia is present in about 70% to 80%,[2] and 10% to 12% have thymoma.[1,2] Significant data exist to support an immunopathologic role of the thymus in the development of

autoimmune MG.[3] First, thymic epithelial cells express low levels of AChR, which is believed to prime naïve helper T cells for autoimmune reactivity. Second, the thymus contains a small number of "myoid" cells, which are the only cells expressing AChR outside muscle in the body. Primed T cells can then recognize these cells to form germinal centers in the hyperplastic thymus and further trigger autoimmunity against AChR.

ROLE OF SURGICAL THERAPY

The beneficial role of surgery for patients with MG was first described by Blalock[4] before the mid-twentieth century. Further clinical reports of the benefits of the thymectomy led to the acceptance of this procedure for patients with generalized MG as a standard of practice. With insight, retrospective studies thereafter suggested that patients undergoing thymectomy had higher remission rates than those treated medically.[5] However, the changes in intensive care unit (ICU) care, ventilatory support, and the introduction of immunosuppressive therapy also have improved the clinical course of this disease and outcomes over time.

Disclosure Statement: The authors have no financial conflict of interest to disclose.

[a] Division of Thoracic Surgery, Toronto General Hospital, University of Toronto, 200 Elizabeth Street 9N-946, Toronto, ON M5G 2C4, Canada; [b] Division of Thoracic Surgery, Innovation, Department of Surgery, University of Toronto, University Health Network, Toronto General Hospital, 200 Elizabeth Street 9N-946, Toronto, ON M5G 2C4, Canada

* Corresponding author.

E-mail address: shaf.keshavjee@uhn.ca

In addition, patient selection and methods of analysis of results varied from center to center, which prevented definitive comparisons. As such, controversies surrounding the role of surgery in the treatment of MG abounded for a long time in the literature, and thymectomy was only considered an option to increase the probability of remission or improvement.

Whatever these historical uncertainties, the benefit of surgical resection in nonthymomatous MG patients has recently been confirmed in the MGTX study, an international, multicenter, randomized trial designed to determine whether thymectomy combined with a standardized immunosuppression protocol would be superior to immunosuppression alone.[6] After 3 years, patients who underwent thymectomy had a significantly lower average quantitative MG score, needed less prednisone or additional immunosuppression, and required fewer hospitalizations for exacerbations. Patients in the thymectomy group also had significantly fewer symptoms related to immunosuppressive medications and lower distress levels related to symptoms, further indicating a better quality of life. The investigators concluded that thymectomy significantly improved clinical outcomes over medical management alone in patients with nonthymomatous MG. The MGTX trial was a landmark in that, for the first time, it compared surgical resection with medical management in a randomized trial and provided level I evidence of the beneficial effect of thymectomy in MG. Surgically, the investigators standardized the study to the transsternal thymectomy, chosen because it provides "reproducible resection of the maximal amount of thymic tissue with low morbidity and a limited risk of phrenic-nerve injury." As described later, less-invasive techniques to resect the thymus gland exist, and several studies have shown equivalence in outcome when maximal procedures via sternotomy were compared with less-invasive approaches.

In terms of postoperative expectations and monitoring, the benefits of thymectomy are often delayed because only 25% of patients achieve remission in the first year, 40% by the end of the second year, and 55% in the third year.[7]

SURGICAL OPTIONS

Thanks to the MGTX study, the point of debate in the surgical treatment of MG can now be definitively transferred the preferred surgical approach. On the one hand, some centers recommend maximal thymectomy via a combined transsternal and transcervical approach (the Jaretzki procedure) to eliminate the gland and any possible extra-anatomical (ectopic) thymic tissue.[8,9] Such an extensive dissection can also be achieved with a standard transsternal approach. On the other hand, thymectomy can be achieved with a minimally invasive transcervical approach, a procedure that was further refined with the introduction of video-assisted (uniportal) transcervical thymectomy. Although the term "uniportal" has become popular in recent years, it should be noted that this approach for thymectomy is not new.[10–12] With the expansion of video-assisted transthoracic surgery (VATS), other thoracoscopic approaches have also gained popularity. Several variations exist, including unilateral, bilateral, bilateral combined with cervical, and robotic procedures. The most recent addition for surgical treatment of MG is the infrasternal (subxiphoid), either thoracoscopic or mediastinoscopic, approach for thymectomy.[13] All procedures allow extracapsular resection of thymus and vary somewhat in the extent of mediastinal fat removed, which may contain ectopic foci of thymic tissue.

Proponents of extended resection advocate the need for maximal approaches to achieve a more complete tissue dissection. However, maximal thymectomy is associated with an increased risk of recurrent and phrenic nerve injury, and ectopic thymic foci are usually limited to 1 or 2 sites, most frequently in the anterior mediastinal fat that can be resected with minimal invasive approaches.[14–16] Of note, the presence of ectopic thymic foci is potentially one of the strongest predictors of poor outcome, even after maximal thymectomy.[17,18] Overall the types of thymectomy have not been directly compared in any randomized study, and outcome data do not support improved results with "maximal thymectomy" over more minimally invasive procedures.[11,12,19] Furthermore, approaches that are more patient-friendly are more easily accepted by the young and female patient population and better tolerated by the older and comorbid patients, and also by neurologists.

To understand the different surgical approaches and categorize the extent of resection of thymus and surrounding tissue, the Myasthenia Gravis Foundation of America has broadly classified varying surgical techniques based on the approach and extent of surgical resection.[20] A meta-analysis of 21 retrospective studies demonstrated a benefit of thymectomy in patients with MG by all types of approach. Furthermore, relatively large case series have shown comparable remission and improvement rates in MG patients with different types of thymectomy.[11,12,19] Thus it is not evident that more extensive thymectomy procedures are more effective. Statistical reshuffling of crude data from different study reports may show different outcomes for different surgical interventions, but this type of reanalysis in itself may produce flawed results and does not provide definitive evidence of the benefits of one surgical approach over another. Ideally, a randomized trial of the different approaches would need to be conducted. Currently no such study is planned and there is no consensus on the optimal surgical approach. Without randomized comparative studies, the decision regarding the surgical approach must rest on the surgeon's individual experience and facility with each given procedure. The underlying principle for thymectomy for MG remains the same regardless of surgical approach: a safe and complete thymectomy.

All patients should have a computed tomography scan of the thorax before surgery to exclude a thymoma. Although VATS seems to be a safe and feasible technique for early-stage thymoma, this approach is controversial and the follow-up times are still short considering that pleural metastases can appear more than 10 years after surgery.[21] Therefore, if a thymoma is present, the preferred surgical approach remains a sternotomy or partial upper sternotomy.

PATIENT SELECTION

Although the current consensus is to use thymectomy for patients with nonthymomatous generalized myasthenia, the role of surgery in other patient groups is much more controversial. In younger patients with ocular MG we recommend surgery at the time of diagnosis, although some clinicians still hesitate to recommend surgery for this group.[22] An important area of debate is the upper age limit for thymectomy. Because older individuals have thymic atrophy rather than hyperplasia, the use of surgery in this group does not seem to have the same theoretic rationale as in younger patients. In addition, one may be concerned that complications of surgery are likely to be greater in older patients. This has to be considered, however, in the context of what can be achieved today with improved anesthesia and minimally invasive techniques for thymectomy, balanced with the ravages of chronic immunosuppression in the elderly population. There are, in fact, retrospective studies reporting that thymectomy is safe in patients older than 60 years, and 16% of those patients over the age of 60 have thymic hyperplasia.[23] Other retrospective series have shown that age does predict outcome in thymectomy for MG, with lower response rates in older subjects.[24] Considering the low morbidity

of transcervical thymectomy in contrast to the morbidity of chronic immunosuppression in the elderly patient, we currently offer thymectomy to patients older than 60 years. At the other end of the age spectrum, thymectomy also is not generally recommended in very young children, although it is sometimes necessary in younger teenagers with severe MG.[25]

PREOPERATIVE AND PERIOPERATIVE CARE

The surgical treatment of MG patients should ideally belong to a dedicated team consisting of a neurologist, thoracic surgeon, and anesthesiologist. After the confirmation of the diagnosis of MG, symptoms should be medically stabilized. Cholinesterase inhibitors are used as the first line of therapy. Prednisone and other immunosuppressive agents are used for persistent symptoms. Steroids are avoided preoperatively, if possible, to avoid the adverse effects on wound healing and infections. Thymectomy is never an emergency, and therefore the patient's strength and respiratory status should be optimized before the well-planned elective surgery. There is no role for urgent thymectomy in patients with myasthenic crisis, as immediate clinical improvement postoperatively should not be expected. Furthermore, surgery in the setting of myasthenic crisis predisposes the patient to a significantly increased risk of postoperative respiratory failure.[26] The likelihood of prolonged mechanical ventilation is increased in patients with severe generalized weakness and/or bulbar symptoms. These patients should first be treated with plasmapheresis before surgery to optimize their condition. High-dose intravenous immunoglobulin is sometimes used as an alternative to plasmapheresis. Because of the short-lived benefits of these treatments, surgery should be planned in the following 2 to 3 weeks. It should be noted that surgery should not be performed before 5 days after plasmapheresis because of possible coagulation abnormalities related to the treatment. Over the years at the Toronto General Hospital we have limited the administration of immunosuppressive therapy before surgery, and preoperative stabilization is most often accomplished with pyridostigmine with the addition of plasmapheresis for the higher-grade myasthenic patients only.

Preoperative anesthetic assessment is of importance. The stabilized state of disease can be confirmed just a couple of days before surgery, allowing safe same-day admission for surgery. Patients should take their morning dose of pyridostigmine ideally immediately before surgery. If surgery is delayed or scheduled for the afternoon, another dose of pyridostigmine is given before surgery. No other premedication is administered. Anesthesia can be safely induced with propofol and fentanyl and maintained with isoflurane and nitrous oxide. Propofol is used in addition to inhaled anesthetics for maintenance of anesthesia. Muscle relaxation is rarely required. In patients for whom prednisone has to be maintained, a steroid stress dose is administered. The aim is routine extubation at the end of surgery.

TECHNIQUE OF VIDEO-ASSISTED UNIPORTAL TRANSCERVICAL THYMECTOMY

Transcervical thymectomy was the approach used for the earliest described thymectomies, but was replaced by the transsternal approach by Blalock and his contemporaries midway through the twentieth century.[4,27] We prefer the video-assisted transcervical thymectomy approach for the treatment of nonthymomatous MG because while being a less-invasive procedure it gives excellent bilateral exposure of the thymus, including the upper and the lower poles, and permits complete thymectomy. Furthermore, unlike transthoracic video-assisted thymectomies, the uniportal transcervical route obviates entry into the pleural spaces, negates the need for chest tubes, provides enhanced exposure in the neck region, and does not require split-lung anesthesia via a double-lumen endotracheal tube. It is an efficient and inexpensive procedure with a one-night hospital stay or same-day discharge, and minimal postoperative pain and discomfort to the patient.

Relative contraindications to a transcervical approach include prior mediastinal surgery and/or irradiation, cervical spine disorder limiting extension of the neck, and a significantly hefty body habitus.

Surgery is performed in the supine position and the patient is positioned with the occiput abutting the top of the operative table. An inflatable bag is placed under the shoulders and inflated to provide good neck extension. Both arms are tucked in at the sides. The neck and full anterior chest is prepped in case a sternotomy is required. A single-lumen endotracheal tube is used and no arterial line is used.

A 5-cm curvilinear incision is made in the skin at the base of the neck, one fingerbreadth above the sternal notch, and extended on each side to the medial border of sternocleidomastoid muscle (**Fig. 1**). This incision is extended through the skin and platysma muscle. Flaps are then developed superiorly to the level of the inferior aspect of the thyroid cartilage, inferiorly to the sternal notch, and laterally up to the anterior aspect of

the sternocleidomastoid muscles. Two Gelpi retractors are then inserted, allowing further dissection in the midline to be carried out. The strap muscles are split vertically in the midline from the bottom of the thyroid isthmus down to the manubrium, where all adherences are cauterized down to the manubrial bone and the cleido-cleido ligament is divided. The strap muscles are then elevated bilaterally to expose the superior poles of the thymus gland, which lie opposed to the posterior surface of the sternothyroid muscles. It is imperative that this be done using careful sharp dissection with meticulous attention to the control of small blood vessels with electrocautery. A bloodless field makes it significantly easier to delineate thymic tissue from fatty tissue in the neck. Each superior pole of the gland is mobilized near the inferior thyroid vein. The upper pole is divided between ties at the point where the thymic tissue terminates. A heavy silk suture, cut long, is placed on each upper pole and used as a "traction" suture to facilitate orientation and traction of the gland (**Fig. 2**). To aid orientation of the specimen, a straight instrument is placed on the suture around the right superior pole, and a curved instrument is placed on the suture around the left superior pole. The superior poles are dissected and pulled up, and the capsule of thymus gland is followed inferiorly to the thoracic inlet.

The retrosternal (retromanubrial) space is digitally cleared to accommodate the placement of the Cooper retractor.[10] The Cooper retractor blade is placed beneath the manubrium to elevate it and open the thoracic inlet (see **Fig. 2**). The inflatable pillow that was placed at the start of the procedure is deflated at this point to further improve the thoracic inlet exposure. Care is taken to make sure that the patient's head is not elevated off the operating table by the sternal retractor. As the Cooper retractor opens the thoracic inlet, ribbon retractors are usually placed on the strap muscles laterally and tied to the Cooper bars using Penrose drains to extend exposure. The surgeon then takes up position at the head of the patient and the assistant on the right side.

We use a 5-mm 30° videothoracoscope (Karl Storz Endoskope, Tuttlingen, Germany) at the right lateral aspect of the neck incision to provide light for direct operating and a video-magnified view of the operating field on a monitor (**Fig. 3**).

The dissection of the gland is carried down into the thorax using primarily blunt dissection with peanuts on long-curved Swedish-DeBakey dissectors. The thymus is first freed anteriorly from the posterior aspect of the sternum until the pericardium is clearly seen at the inferior edge of the

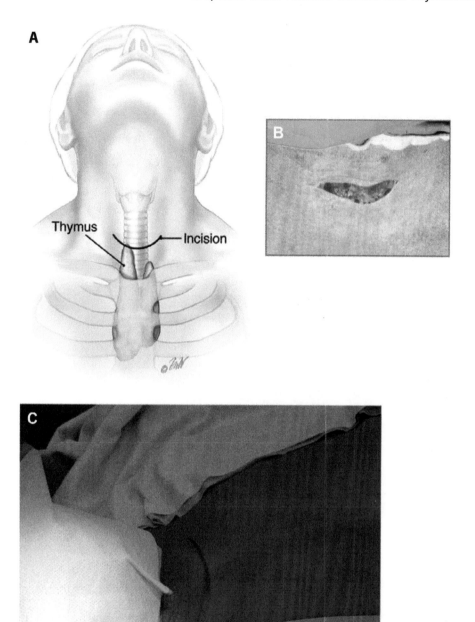

Fig. 1. An incision is made in the skin at the base of the neck, one fingerbreadth above the sternal notch, and extended on each side to the medial border of sternocleidomastoid muscle. (*A*) Representation of the incision with respect to upper poles of the thymus. (*B*) Skin incision at the base of the neck, one finger breath above the sternal notch. (*C*) To avoid distorsion, the incision site is first marked at the skin. (*From* Sihvo E, Keshavjee S. Transcervical thymectomy. In: Sugarbaker DJ, Bueno R, Colson YL, et al. Adult chest surgery. 2nd edition. New York: McGraw-Hill; 2015. p. 1256; with permission.)

gland on the midline (**Fig. 4**). The dissection of the gland is then carried out laterally on both sides until the inferior poles are clearly identified. The dissector is placed on the pericardium, distal to the inferior pole of the thymus, and in a sweeping motion the gland is extracted from the inferior mediastinum. Once fully mobilized anteriorly, the upper pole stay-sutures are retracted anteriorly over the cross bar of the Cooper retractor to bring the thymus up to the sternum and allow posterior

A

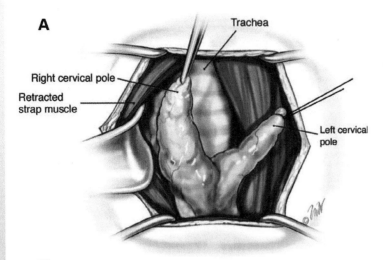

Trachea

Right cervical pole

Retracted
strap muscle

Left cervical
pole

B

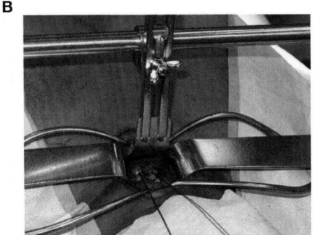

Fig. 2. Dissection of the upper poles of the thymus and placement of the Copper retractor. A: Representation of the dissected upper poles of the thymus. B: Cooper retractor is in place. Traction sutures are placed on each upper pole of the thymus gland. (*From* Sihvo E, Keshavjee S. Transcervical thymectomy. In: Sugarbaker DJ, Bueno R, Colson YL, et al. Adult chest surgery. 2nd edition. New York: McGraw-Hill; 2015. p. 1257; with permission.)

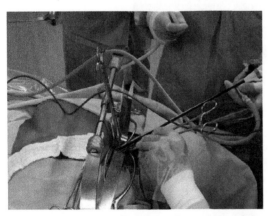

Fig. 3. Operative view illustrating the position of the telescope and instruments through the cervical incision. (*From* Sihvo E, Keshavjee S. Transcervical thymectomy. In: Sugarbaker DJ, Bueno R, Colson YL, et al. Adult chest surgery. 2nd edition. New York: McGraw-Hill; 2015. p. 1257; with permission.)

dissection of the gland off of the innominate vein and pericardium posteriorly (**Fig. 5**). The arterial vessels entering the gland laterally from the internal thoracic artery branches are clipped with stainless-steel clips. The thymic veins (there are often several), which drain into the innominate vein, are identified posteriorly and divided between stainless-steel clips. The assistance of the videothoracoscope provides good visualization of the lower mediastinum, down to the diaphragm.

The ventilation rate and tidal volume are both decreased, or even intermittently held when needed, to facilitate exposure in the mediastinum. A 7 Jackson-Pratt drain (Zimmer, Dover, OH) is usually inserted through a lateral stab wound in the neck and placed down into the mediastinum, and the Cooper retractor is removed. The strap muscles are approximated, and the platysma and the skin are closed. Patients are discharged

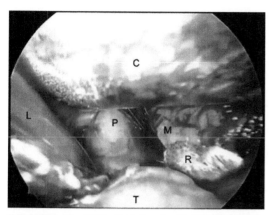

Fig. 4. The thymus is first freed anteriorly from the manubrium using peanuts on Swedish-DeBakey forceps, until pericardium is seen in the midline. Dissection is then carried out laterally to the right then left inferior poles of the gland using a combination of blunt and sharp dissection. C, Cooper retractor; L, left Swedish-DeBackey with peanut; P, pericardium; M, mediastinal fat; R, right Swedish-DeBackey with peanut; T, thymus gland.

home on the morning after surgery. A video of this procedure is available online (http://www.asvide.com/articles/724).[28]

In rare instances, if complete thymectomy cannot be performed through the transcervical route, the operation can be converted to a partial upper sternotomy. This is carried out by the addition of a vertical skin incision extending down from the sternal notch onto the upper sternum. The sternum is then divided with the oscillating saw, extending laterally in the third intercostal space (unilaterally in a "J" or bilaterally in a "T") to create

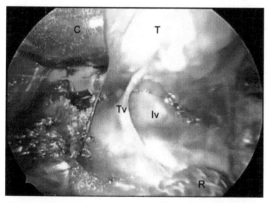

Fig. 5. After complete anterior dissection, the thymus is reflected anteriorly to complete the posterior dissection over the innominate vein, allowing identification, dissection, and clipping of the thymic veins. C, Cooper retractor; T, thymus gland; Iv, innominate vein; Tv, thymic vein; R, right Swedish-DeBackey with peanut.

a partial upper sternotomy, which provides sufficient exposure to easily complete the operation.

Postoperative Care

The patient's respiratory status and requirements for ventilatory support are, by far, the most salient issues in the postoperative period. With careful preoperative preparation of the MG patient, ventilatory issues are rarely a problem. Patients are extubated in the operating room. They are instructed to take their morning dose of anticholinesterase medication with a sip of water immediately preoperatively, to optimize their strength at the time of extubation, and are given an additional dose in the recovery room. With the minimally invasive approach, the need for postoperative analgesia can be limited to acetaminophen with mild narcotics such as codeine. Strong narcotics are rarely required. Oral pyridostigmine at the patient's usual dose is resumed 4 to 6 hours after surgery. If patients are on steroid therapy before surgery, oral steroids are continued at the patient's usual dose the next morning. With minimally invasive approaches today, patients almost never need postoperative care in the ICU and are ready to be discharged later in the day or early the next morning.

MG medications are not altered until 6 weeks after surgery when they are seen by the surgeon and the neurologist. A period of 3 to 12 months is most often observed before clinical improvement can be seen following thymectomy.[14] Some patients may improve in a few weeks whereas some become transiently worse postoperatively. Myasthenic exacerbation, rather than surgical considerations, is the usual reason to keep a patient in the hospital for longer than 1 day. If symptoms worsen, the medication regimen may have to be altered to include prednisone or azathioprine. An occasional patient may deteriorate considerably into myasthenic crisis. These patients should be expediently treated with plasmapheresis to prevent deterioration to the point of requiring ventilatory support.

Procedure-Specific Complications

The rate of surgical complications is low, less than 2% in our series.[11] These were hemothorax and pneumothorax, treated successfully by conservative methods. Wound complications have also been reported. The rate of recurrent nerve injuries is zero. The reported conversion rate is now in the range of 1%.[11,29]

SUMMARY

The uniportal video-assisted transcervical technique offers a minimally invasive surgical approach with a low complication rate, a good cosmetic result, and a short length of recovery for a complete thymectomy in patients with MG. Patient acceptance with this less-invasive technique is better, leading to greater application of surgery earlier in the course of the disease.

REFERENCES

1. Gilhus NE. Myasthenia gravis. N Engl J Med 2017; 376(13):e25.
2. Hohlfeld R, Wekerle H. The role of the thymus in myasthenia gravis. Adv Neuroimmunol 1994;4(4):373–86.
3. Luo J, Kuryatov A, Lindstrom JM. Specific immunotherapy of experimental myasthenia gravis by a novel mechanism. Ann Neurol 2010;67(4):441–51.
4. Blalock A. Thymectomy in the treatment of myasthenia gravis. report of twenty cases. J Thorac Surg 1944;13:316.
5. Mantegazza R, Baggi F, Antozzi C, et al. Myasthenia gravis (MG): epidemiological data and prognostic factors. Ann N Y Acad Sci 2003;998:413–23.
6. Wolfe GI, Kaminski HJ, Aban IB, et al. Randomized trial of thymectomy in myasthenia gravis. N Engl J Med 2016;375(6):511–22.
7. Perlo VP, Arnason B, Poskanzer D, et al. The role of thymectomy in the treatment of myasthenia gravis. Ann N Y Acad Sci 1971;183:308–15.
8. Jaretzki A 3rd, Wolff M. "Maximal" thymectomy for myasthenia gravis. Surgical anatomy and operative technique. J Thorac Cardiovasc Surg 1988;96(5): 711–6.
9. Jaretzki A, Steinglass KM, Sonett JR. Thymectomy in the management of myasthenia gravis. Semin Neurol 2004;24(1):49–62.
10. Cooper JD, Al-Jilaihawa AN, Pearson FG, et al. An improved technique to facilitate transcervical thymectomy for myasthenia gravis. Ann Thorac Surg 1988;45(3):242–7.
11. de Perrot M, Bril V, McRae K, et al. Impact of minimally invasive trans-cervical thymectomy on outcome in patients with myasthenia gravis. Eur J Cardiothorac Surg 2003;24(5):677–83.
12. Zahid I, Sharif S, Routledge T, et al. Video-assisted thoracoscopic surgery or transsternal thymectomy in the treatment of myasthenia gravis? Interact Cardiovasc Thorac Surg 2011;12(1):40–6.
13. Murai H, Uchiyama A, Mei FJ, et al. Long-term effects of infrasternal mediastinoscopic thymectomy in myasthenia gravis. J Neurol Sci 2009;287(1–2):185–7.
14. Bulkley GB, Bass KN, Stephenson GR, et al. Extended cervicomediastinal thymectomy in the integrated management of myasthenia gravis. Ann Surg 1997;226(3):324–34 [discussion: 334–5].
15. Fukai I, Funato Y, Mizuno T, et al. Distribution of thymic tissue in the mediastinal adipose tissue. J Thorac Cardiovasc Surg 1991;101(6):1099–102.
16. Klimek-Piotrowska W, Mizia E, Kuzdzal J, et al. Ectopic thymic tissue in the mediastinum: limitations for the operative treatment of myasthenia gravis. Eur J Cardiothorac Surg 2012;42(1):61–5.
17. Ambrogi V, Mineo TC. Active ectopic thymus predicts poor outcome after thymectomy in class III myasthenia gravis. J Thorac Cardiovasc Surg 2012;143(3):601–6.
18. Ozdemir N, Kara M, Dikmen E, et al. Predictors of clinical outcome following extended thymectomy in myasthenia gravis. Eur J Cardiothorac Surg 2003; 23(2):233–7.
19. Meyer DM, Herbert MA, Sobhani NC, et al. Comparative clinical outcomes of thymectomy for myasthenia gravis performed by extended transsternal and minimally invasive approaches. Ann Thorac Surg 2009;87(2):385–90 [discussion: 390–1].
20. Gronseth GS, Barohn RJ. Practice parameter: thymectomy for autoimmune myasthenia gravis (an evidence-based review): report of the Quality Standards Subcommittee of the American Academy of Neurology. Neurology 2000;55(1):7–15.
21. Pennathur A, Qureshi I, Schuchert MJ, et al. Comparison of surgical techniques for early-stage thymoma: feasibility of minimally invasive thymectomy and comparison with open resection. J Thorac Cardiovasc Surg 2011;141(3):694–701.
22. Benatar M, Kaminski HJ, Quality Standards Subcommittee of the American Academy of Neurology. Evidence report: the medical treatment of ocular myasthenia (an evidence-based review): report of the Quality Standards Subcommittee of the American Academy of Neurology. Neurology 2007; 68(24):2144–9.
23. Tsuchida M, Yamato Y, Souma T, et al. Efficacy and safety of extended thymectomy for elderly patients with myasthenia gravis. Ann Thorac Surg 1999; 67(6):1563–7.
24. Budde JM, Morris CD, Gal AA, et al. Predictors of outcome in thymectomy for myasthenia gravis. Ann Thorac Surg 2001;72(1):197–202.
25. Evoli A. Acquired myasthenia gravis in childhood. Curr Opin Neurol 2010;23(5):536–40.
26. Gracey DR, Divertie MB, Howard FM Jr, et al. Postoperative respiratory care after transsternal thymectomy in myasthenia gravis. A 3-year experience in 53 patients. Chest 1984;86(1):67–71.
27. Schumacher ED, Roth J. Thymecktomie bei einem Fall von Murbus Basedowii mit Myasthenie. Mitt Grenzgeb Med Chir (Jena) 1912;25: 746–65.
28. Donahoe L, Keshavjee S. Video-assisted transcervical thymectomy for myasthenia gravis. Ann Cardiothorac Surg 2015;4(6):561–3.
29. Shrager JB. Extended transcervical thymectomy: the ultimate minimally invasive approach. Ann Thorac Surg 2010;89(6):S2128–34.

Technique for Myasthenia Gravis: Subxiphoid Approach

Beatrice Aramini, MD, PhD[a], Jiang Fan, MD, PhD[b],*

KEYWORDS

- Subxiphoid thymectomy • Myasthenia gravis • VATS thymectomy • Minimally invasive surgery
- Open thymectomy • Sternotomy

KEY POINTS

- Surgical resection of thymoma has been recommended as the principal treatment, and complete-ness of resection is considered the most important determinant of the long-term survival in thymomas.
- Recent studies have reported thymectomy for myasthenia gravis and anterior mediastinal tumors using a minimally invasive approach rather than conventional median sternotomy.
- Video-assisted thoracic surgery (VATS) is widely used in thoracic surgery for anterior mediastinal tumors or myasthenia gravis (MG).
- The subxiphoid approach led to less-invasive thymectomy and extended the indications for VATS for invasive anterior mediastinal tumors.
- The subxiphoid approach improves patient satisfaction, reduces pain, and offers superior aesthetic outcomes.

 Video content accompanies this article at http://www.thoracic.theclinics.com

INTRODUCTION

Currently, surgical techniques that are less inva-sive than conventional median sternotomy are used for thymectomy in the treatment of myasthenia gravis (MG) and anterior mediastinal tumors, so no sternal incision is required (Videos 1–4).[1–8] Among the minimally invasive ap-proaches, 3 are widely used for thymectomy. Although the first thymectomy was performed transcervically by Sauerbruch in 1912,[9] trans-sternal access gained popularity in the 1980s following the results of Jaretzki and colleagues,[10] who recommended a "maximal transcervical-trans-sternal thymectomy" for non-thymomatous MG patients. Since then, the trans-sternal approach has been used and described with different modifications.[11] In 1988, Cooper and col-leagues[12] described an extended transcervical approach using a dedicated self-retaining sternal retractor to lift the sternum. This technique offered the advantage of causing minimal pain because it does not involve access through the intercostal space. However, the surgical operability and field of view are very poor; thus, this technique is not widely used.[13] The second approach is *lateral tho-racotomy*, which is currently the most widely used technique, especially for large anterior mediastinal masses or infiltrating tumors. Even if the traditional approach to thymectomy by median sternotomy or lateral thoracotomy is based on the assumption that it is the best means to achieve adequate

---

Disclosure Statement: The authors have nothing to disclose.
 a Division of Thoracic Surgery, Department of Medical and Surgical Sciences for Children and Adults, University of Modena and Reggio Emilia, Modena 41124, Italy; b Department of Thoracic Surgery, Shanghai Pulmonary Hospital, Tongji University School of Medicine, Shanghai 200433, China
* Corresponding author.
E-mail address: drjiangfan@yahoo.com

Thorac Surg Clin 29 (2019) 195–202
https://doi.org/10.1016/j.thorsurg.2018.12.010

resection margins, complete removal of the thymus and clearance of the anterior mediastinal fat, Landreneau and colleagues[14] in 1992 removed an anterior mediastinal tumor under thoracoscopy. Recently, *video-assisted thoracoscopic surgery (VATS) thymectomy* has been gaining acceptance as a means to achieve adequate oncologic results and symptomatic improvement of myasthenic symptoms with less impact on the patient. This approach is also commonly used in robot-assisted thymectomy.[15,16]

The third minimally invasive technique reported by Kido and colleagues[17] in 1999 is the *subxiphoid approach*. This approach offers a better view from the midline of the body that permits identification of the location of the superior pole of the thymus and bilateral phrenic nerves. This approach avoids intercostal nerve damage with minimal pain and excellent cosmetic outcomes.

Various surgical modifications currently used for thymectomy have been suggested.[18–23]

SURGICAL TECHNIQUE
Pre-operative Planning

Patient selection for the subxiphoid VATS thymectomy approach is recommended based on the good field of view provided this procedure, which is indicated in patients with MG and/or anterior mediastinal tumors who do not require surgical suturing. In the event that the mass infiltrates anatomic structures that require more attention and working space, that is, pericardium infiltration, additional ports or open surgery should be considered. However, for advanced operable stages, especially after radiation therapy, median sternotomy, or lateral thoracotomy should be planned.

Computerized tomographic (CT) scanning is routinely performed in patients before surgery and after tumor resection to screen for thymoma recurrence. If MG or other symptoms arises, CT could be the first choice (**Fig. 1**). However, CT is a morphologic examination; before surgery, patients with anterior mediastinal mass should undergo physical and neurologic examination, electromyography, and acetylcholine receptor antibody blood test.

Positron emission tomography (PET)-CT could compensate for the limitations of CT by measuring the metabolic rate of tissue, which improves the diagnostic accuracy. The overall sensitivity of CT for detecting the mediastinal recurrence and pleural dissemination of thymomas is 71%, and its specificity is 85%. Regarding PET-CT, the overall sensitivity and specificity for thymoma recurrence are 82% and 95%, respectively.[24]

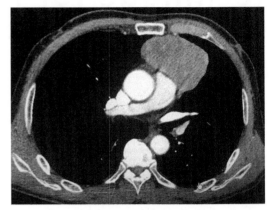

Fig. 1. CT scan reveals an anterior mediastinal tumor with no infiltration signs.

Magnetic resonance imaging is a method that uses a low radiation dose and better represents cystic tissue than CT. Magnetic resonance imaging offers advantages for differentiating thymic hyperplasia and thymoma and evaluating whether the phrenic nerve is infiltrated.[25]

Preparation and Patient Positioning

The patient is placed in the supine position (**Fig. 2**). The operator stands between the patient's legs and the surgical assistant with the camera stands to the right of the patient to operate the 30° camera scope. A monitor is positioned at the patient's head (**Fig. 3**).

Mechanical ventilation with a double-lumen endotracheal tube is used, with the patient under general anesthesia for one-lung ventilation. The peripheral intravenous drip route is secured to the right upper or lower limb, making it possible to clamp the innominate vein in the event of injury to this vein.

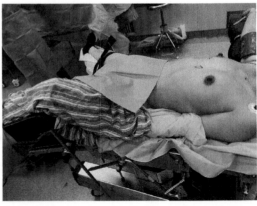

Fig. 2. Patient preparation before surgery.

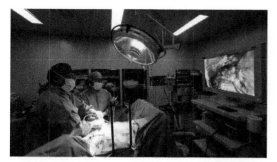

Fig. 3. Surgeon and operative room during subxiphoid thymectomy.

Surgical Approach

A vertical 4-cm skin incision approximately 1-cm caudal to the xiphoid process (**Fig. 4**A), and an additional 2-cm skin incision between the fourth and fifth intercostal anterior axillary line on the right side, are used for camera placement; these surgical access points are used at the end of the operation for the placement of chest drains (**Fig. 4**B). A surgical assistant is typically placed to the right of the patient; however, the camera may be moved to the other side if necessary (**Fig. 5**A). A 1-cm incision is generated for the placement of hooks, which are tightened by 2 retractors (**Fig. 5**B, C).

SURGICAL PROCEDURE
Step 1: Surgical Access

Caution should be exercised given that it can be difficult for the forceps to reach the posterior aspect of the sternum if the skin incision is made too close to the xiphoid process. To guarantee

better access and exposure of the anatomic structures in the anterior mediastinum, a hook is placed at the level of the jugular process behind the manubrium of the sternum, and another hook is placed behind of the lower portion of the sternum after resection of the subxiphoid process. Thereafter, a 4-cm vertical incision is made on the fascia of the rectus abdominis without opening the peritoneum, and a space is created to insert the port. An Alexis wound retractor (Applied Medical, Rancho Santa Margherita, CA, USA) is used to protect the access during the operation (**Fig. 6**). There is no need to dissect the xiphoid process.

Step 2: Thymus Isolation

The surgeon detaches the thymus from the posterior aspect of the sternum to the neck using the HARMONIC ACE+7 (Ethicon, Cincinnati, OH, USA) device. Bilateral incisions are generated in the mediastinal pleura, and the thoracic cavity is exposed bilaterally. Next, the locations of the bilateral phrenic nerves are identified. The location of the left phrenic nerve on the caudal side in the thoracic cavity can be verified by either pulling the pericardial adipose tissue to the right or by displacing the heart with cotton swabs for thoracoscopic surgery. The pericardial adipose tissue and thymus are detached from the pericardium in an anterior manner from the bilateral phrenic nerves. To prevent collateral damage to the adjacent organs when using a vessel-sealing device, the device should be used only once the dissected thymus is at a safe distance and is sufficiently detached from vital structures, such as the pericardium and brachiocephalic vein. The surgeon

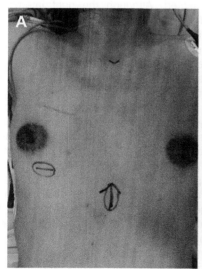
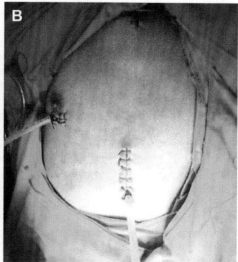

Fig. 4. (*A*) Surgical ports access is established before the operation. (*B*) Chest drain placement after surgery.

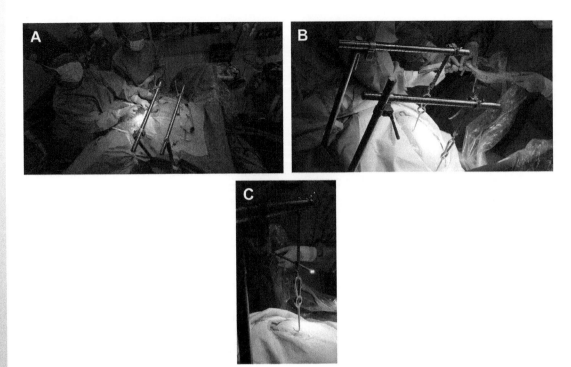

Fig. 5. Hooks are inserted in the jugular and subxiphoid incision and tightened by 2 retractors (*A*, *B*). Hooks and 30° camera (*C*).

proceeds along the innominate vein with the closure of the thymic veins (1–5 thymic veins are typically noted) with vascular clips (hemlock) until the left internal thoracic vein (left mammary vein) is visualized. The dissection proceeds cranially with closure and division of the lower thyroid veins in the same manner as that used for thymic veins. The dissection further proceeds along thymic poles (horns) until the lower portion of the thyroid is clearly visualized. During the dissection, structures, such as the innominate, the brachiocephalic trunk artery, the common carotid, and the trachea, are always visualized. The laryngeal recurrent and vagus nerves are preserved.

The left lobe of the thymus is pulled toward the right of the patient by bending the forceps of the left hand to the right. At this point, the surgeon crosses hands to detach the left lobe with the HARMONIC device (Ethicon). The right lobe of the thymus is pulled toward the left of the patient by bending the forceps to the left. The surgeon does not need to cross hands for this step. The lower pole of the thymus is detached from the pericardium. A trick to perform this surgery well is to firmly grasp the thymus near the detachment site with the forceps in the left hand and pull. To safely expose the distal side of the left brachiocephalic vein, the superficial adipose tissue is slowly and gradually detached from the area near the left brachiocephalic vein. The proximal side of the left

brachiocephalic vein is close to where this vein joins the right internal thoracic vein. Similar to the distal side, the proximal side is exposed by slowly and gradually detaching superficial adipose tissue from the area thought to be near the left brachiocephalic vein. Once the proximal side of the left brachiocephalic vein is exposed, the area of the confluence of the brachiocephalic veins is exposed. Thereafter, the neck portion is detached, and the thin membrane above the thymus is dissected. Although the right internal thoracic vein is not typically dissected, it can be dissected if it hinders the operation. Although exercising caution to not injure the left brachiocephalic vein, the superior pole of the thymus is grasped using grasper forceps and pulled caudally to push the left brachiocephalic vein and expose a good field of vision of the neck. The superior pole of the thymus and the cervical adipose tissue are dissected from the right brachiocephalic vein on the right side, the thyroid at the upper end, the brachiocephalic artery and trachea on the posterior aspect, and the left brachiocephalic vein on the left side. Due care should be exercised to not damage the inferior thyroid vein. Finally, the thymus is pulled to either the right or left and dissected from the innominate vein. In the sequential order of the procedure, the thymic vein is dissected using the HARMONIC device, and thymectomy is completed. The liberated upper horns of the

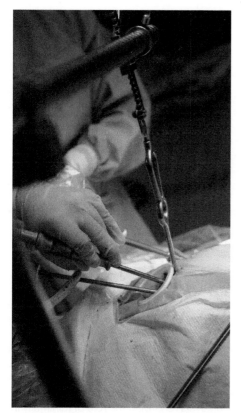

Fig. 6. A wound retractor is placed through the subxiphoid incision.

thymus are grasped and pulled caudally, enabling dissection of the thymus from the pericardium and the left mediastinal pleura, which is partially resected. Finally, the thymus is pulled to either the right or left and dissected from the innominate vein (**Fig. 7**). The thymus is finally placed in the plastic bag and removed through the subxiphoid incision (**Fig. 8**). Dissection of the aorta-pulmonary window is completed. Hemostasis is

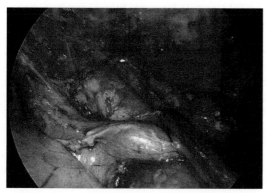

Fig. 7. Left innominate vein and left mammary vein after thymectomy. The left pleura is partially opened.

assessed. VATS ports are removed. The resected thymus is placed in an endobag in the mediastinum and removed from the body through the subxiphoid incision. Two chest drains (variable from 20Fr to 28Fr, depending of the patient's size) are placed, 1 inserted through the subxiphoid incision in the left thoracic cavity and 1 inserted through the right access in the right pleural space, or both into the subxiphoid incision, and the surgical incision is closed.

Immediate Postoperative Care

After surgery, patients with no complications are monitored in the thoracic surgery unit. A chest radiograph and blood test are performed on the day of the operation. Patients with a preoperative MG diagnosis are placed preventively in the intensive care unit for 24 hours. The chest drainage is removed the day after surgery. Patients are typically discharged from the hospital after 2 to 3 days.

Rehabilitation and Recovery

Patients are typically assessed 1 week after surgery and undergo chest radiography. Follow-up for thymoma and thymic carcinoma is set by current guidelines.[26]

In our surgical experience, the mean observation period after thymectomy for thymoma was 10.1 months (range: 0.5–26.0 months after operation). No mortality was reported in this period.

CLINICAL RESULTS IN THE LITERATURE

Thymectomy is recommended for the treatment of thymoma. Surgical resection for thymoma is regarded as the principal treatment, and the completeness of resection is considered to be the most important determinant of the long-term survival of the patients with thymomas.[27,28]

In recent years, minimally invasive approaches have replaced conventional median sternotomy in thymectomy for thymoma or MG.[29]

VATS thymectomy for MG and anterior mediastinal tumors was initially reported in the early 1990s.[17,27,28,30,31] Although sternal wound complications occasionally become problematic following sternotomy, the incidence of sternal wound complications disappeared with the use of VATS thymectomy.[31–33] Although many groups have reported on the use of VATS thymectomy, the technique is not widespread based on the following hypothesized reasons. First, the thymus is surrounded by the sternum, the pericardium, and the pleura. Median sternotomy has been used for thymectomy for many years.[12,14,29]

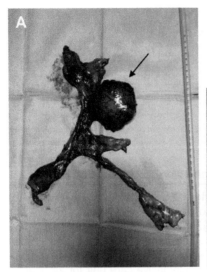
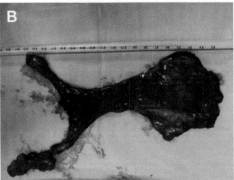

Fig. 8. Thymoma and thymus gland (*A, B*).

Many thoracic surgeons prefer sternotomy for thymectomy even if they often perform VATS operations for lung cancer. This notion could be justified based on the following reasons. Surgeons prefer to understand the anatomy of the mediastinum from the viewpoint of median sternotomy. The working space is severely limited owing to the position of the thymus, which is a gland surrounded by many organs. In addition, difficulties in the operative procedures potentially influence the use of the technique.

To overcome such difficulties, the subxiphoid approach has been used in recent years.[13,18,20,29,34,35] This technique offers the following advantages: the view is similar to the view from median sternotomy and the view looking-up from the main incision using this approach is familiar to thoracic surgeons. Second, to overcome the challenge of the working space, many surgeons have increased the working spaces by lifting the sternum or using CO_2 insufflation, which beneficially compress all organs and structures, thus securing the space from the sternum to the heart.[36,37]

The subxiphoid approach is not more widely used because thoracic surgeons are unfamiliar with this approach. One of the main complications during this surgery is bleeding of the main vessels. The response to that is vital, and countermeasures for bleeding from the innominate vein are important in thymectomy. If bleeding occurs, the first step is to stop the bleeding by applying pressure using the thymus or a swab for thoracoscopy. An attempt should be made to stop the bleeding by applying a fibrin sheet or other hemostatic agents to the bleeding point. If these methods do not stop

the bleeding, the surgeon should promptly switch to median sternotomy, which is easy given that a subxiphoid approach is performed with the patient in a supine position. However, experience with this technique is mandatory.[37] In 2016, Friedant and colleagues[38] published a systematic review and meta-analysis regarding the role of minimally invasive versus open thymectomy for thymic malignancies and reported no statistically significant differences in overall R0 resections for the minimally invasive surgery (MIS) or open groups; however, the trend favored patients in the MIS group. The only statistically significant clinical outcomes observed were decreased blood loss and reduced length of hospital stay, both of which favored the minimally invasive group. No differences in operating time or complications were noted between the 2 groups.

SUMMARY

Current literature suggests that minimally invasive surgery may be as effective as or better than open thymectomy in treating small, early-stage thymic malignancies.[24,25,39–44] Studies have reported comparable survival data and oncologic outcomes between the 2 procedures[19–21]; however, such claims are limited by the small sample size and lack of long-term follow-up comparisons between patients who underwent MIS and those who underwent open thymectomy.

There are 2 main advantages of the subxiphoid approach: the reduction of pain after surgery and the aesthetic result. Furthermore, the subxiphoid approach uses only 1 or 2 ports for access. In fact, this technique avoids intercostal nerve damage due to the subxiphoid access, and the eventual small collateral incision. Suda and colleagues[13,34] in 2016 published a description of monoportal VATS suxiphoid thymectomy and "*multiple-ports*" robotic subxiphoid thymectomy. Further steps need to be set to develop a future single-port robotic thymectomy through the subxiphoid access. However, this technique is recommended for small- to middle-sized anterior mediastinal tumors, possibly without infiltration of the main vessels and the surrounding structures. Recently, an increased incidence has been noted for small-sized anterior mediastinal tumors. This increase is presumably associated with the combination of increased radiological procedures with medical examinations.

SUPPLEMENTARY DATA

Supplementary data to this article can be found online at https://doi.org/10.1016/j.thorsurg.2018.12.010.

REFERENCES

1. Venuta F, Anile M, Diso D, et al. Thymoma and thymic carcinoma. Eur J Cardiothorac Surg 2010; 37(1):13–25.

2. Spaggiari L, Casiraghi M, Guarize J. Multidisciplinary treatment of malignant thymoma. Curr Opin Oncol 2012;24(2):117–22.

3. Detterbeck FC, Parsons AM. Thymic tumors. Ann Thorac Surg 2004;77(5):1860–9.

4. Jaretzki A 3rd, Sonett JR. Evaluation of results of thymectomy for MG requires accepted standards. Ann Thorac Surg 2007;84(1):360–1 [author reply: 361].

5. Sonett JR, Jaretzki A 3rd. Thymectomy for nonthymomatous myasthenia gravis: a critical analysis. Ann N Y Acad Sci 2008;1132:315–28.

6. Mao ZF, Mo XA, Qin C, et al. Incidence of thymoma in myasthenia gravis: a systematic review. J Clin Neurol 2012;8(3):161–9.

7. Levine GD, Rosai J. Thymic hyperplasia and neoplasia: a review of current concepts. Hum Pathol 1978;9(5):495–515.

8. Ruckert JC, Walter M, Muller JM. Pulmonary function after thoracoscopic thymectomy versus median sternotomy for myasthenia gravis. Ann Thorac Surg 2000;70(5):1656–61.

9. Schumacher E, Roth J. Thymectomy for nonthymomatous myasthenia gravis: a critical analysis. Ann N Y Acad Sci 2008;1132:315–28.

10. Jaretzki A 3rd, Penn AS, Younger DS, et al. "Maximal" thymectomy for myasthenia gravis. Results. J Thorac Cardiovasc Surg 1988;95(5):747–57.

11. Prokakis C, Koletsis E, Salakou S, et al. Modified maximal thymectomy for myasthenia gravis: effect of maximal resection on late neurologic outcome and predictors of disease remission. Ann Thorac Surg 2009;88(5):1638–45.

12. Cooper JD, Al-Jilaihawa AN, Pearson FG, et al. An improved technique to facilitate transcervical thymectomy for myasthenia gravis. Ann Thorac Surg 1988;45(3):242–7.

13. Suda T. Subxiphoid thymectomy: single-port, dual-port, and robot-assisted. J Vis Surg 2017;3:75.

14. Landreneau RJ, Dowling RD, Castillo WM, et al. Thoracoscopic resection of an anterior mediastinal tumor. Ann Thorac Surg 1992;54(1):142–4.

15. Detterbeck F, Youssef S, Ruffini E, et al. A review of prognostic factors in thymic malignancies. J Thorac Oncol 2011;6(7 Suppl 3):S1698–704.

16. Margaritora S, Cesario A, Cusumano G, et al. Thirty-five-year follow-up analysis of clinical and pathologic outcomes of thymoma surgery. Ann Thorac Surg 2010;89(1):245–52 [discussion: 252].

17. Kido T, Hazama K, Inoue Y, et al. Resection of anterior mediastinal masses through an infrasternal approach. Ann Thorac Surg 1999;67(1):263–5.

18. Fang W, Yao X, Antonicelli A, et al. Comparison of surgical approach and extent of resection for Masaoka-Koga stage I and II thymic tumours in Europe, North America and Asia: an international thymic malignancy interest group retrospective database analysis. Eur J Cardiothorac Surg 2017; 52(1):26–32.

19. Sakamaki Y, Oda T, Kanazawa G, et al. Intermediate-term oncologic outcomes after video-assisted thoracoscopic thymectomy for early-stage thymoma. J Thorac Cardiovasc Surg 2014;148(4): 1230–7.e1.

20. Liu TJ, Lin MW, Hsieh MS, et al. Video-assisted thoracoscopic surgical thymectomy to treat early thymoma: a comparison with the conventional transsternal approach. Ann Surg Oncol 2014;21(1): 322–8.

21. Manoly I, Whistance RN, Sreekumar R, et al. Early and mid-term outcomes of trans-sternal and video-assisted thoracoscopic surgery for thymoma. Eur J Cardiothorac Surg 2014;45(6):e187–93.

22. Ye B, Tantai JC, Ge XX, et al. Surgical techniques for early-stage thymoma: video-assisted thoracoscopic thymectomy versus transsternal thymectomy. J Thorac Cardiovasc Surg 2014;147(5):1599–603.

23. Zhao Y, Shi J, Fan L, et al. Surgical treatment of thymoma: an 11-year experience with 761 patients. Eur J Cardiothorac Surg 2016;49(4):1144–9.

24. El-Bawab HY, Abouzied MM, Rafay MA, et al. Clinical use of combined positron emission tomography and computed tomography in thymoma recurrence. Interact Cardiovasc Thorac Surg 2010;11(4):395–9.

25. Carter BW, Benveniste MF, Truong MT, et al. State of the art: MR imaging of thymoma. Magn Reson Imaging Clin N Am 2015;23(2):165–77.

26. Girard N, Ruffini E, Marx A, et al. Thymic epithelial tumours: ESMO clinical practice guidelines for diagnosis, treatment and follow-up. Ann Oncol 2015; 26(Suppl 5):v40–55.

27. Masaoka A, Monden Y, Nakahara K, et al. Follow-up study of thymomas with special reference to their clinical stages. Cancer 1981;48(11):2485–92.

28. Ruckert JC, Swierzy M, Ismail M. Comparison of robotic and nonrobotic thoracoscopic thymectomy: a cohort study. J Thorac Cardiovasc Surg 2011; 141(3):673–7.

29. Detterbeck FC, Kim AW, Zielinski M. Looking in from above and up from below: new vistas in thoracic surgery. Innovations (Phila) 2012;7(3):161–4.

30. Suda T, Sugimura H, Tochii D, et al. Single-port thymectomy through an infrasternal approach. Ann Thorac Surg 2012;93(1):334–6.

31. Kehlet H, Jensen TS, Woolf CJ. Persistent postsurgical pain: risk factors and prevention. Lancet 2006;367(9522):1618–25.

32. Suda T, Tochii D, Tochii S, et al. Trans-subxiphoid robotic thymectomy. Interact Cardiovasc Thorac Surg 2015;20(5):669–71.

33. Suda T. Robotic subxiphoid thymectomy. J Vis Surg 2016;2:118.

34. Suda T, Hachimaru A, Tochii D, et al. Video-assisted thoracoscopic thymectomy versus subxiphoid single-port thymectomy: initial resultsdagger. Eur J Cardiothorac Surg 2016;49(Suppl 1):i54–8.

35. Pennathur A, Qureshi I, Schuchert MJ, et al. Comparison of surgical techniques for early-stage thymoma: feasibility of minimally invasive thymectomy and comparison with open resection. J Thorac Cardiovasc Surg 2011;141(3):694–701.

36. Suda T. Subxiphoid single-port thymectomy in a patient with mature teratoma. Asvide;4(219). Available at: http://www.asvide.com/articles/1529.

37. Suda T. Using a dual-port system eliminates interference between forceps. Asvide 2017;4(220). Available at: http://www.asvide.com/articles/1530.

38. Friedant AJ, Handorf EA, Su S, et al. Minimally invasive versus open thymectomy for thymic malignancies: systematic review and meta-analysis. J Thorac Oncol 2016;11(1):30–8.

39. Tseng YC, Hsieh CC, Huang HY, et al. Is thymectomy necessary in nonmyasthenic patients with early thymoma? J Thorac Oncol 2013;8(7): 952–8.

40. Toker A, Erus S, Ziyade S, et al. It is feasible to operate on pathological Masaoka stage I and II thymoma patients with video-assisted thoracoscopy: analysis of factors for a successful resection. Surg Endosc 2013;27(5):1555–60.

41. Gu ZT, Mao T, Chen WH, et al. Comparison of video-assisted thoracoscopic surgery and median sternotomy approaches for thymic tumor resections at a single institution. Surg Laparosc Endosc Percutan Tech 2015;25(1):47–51.

42. Jurado J, Javidfar J, Newmark A, et al. Minimally invasive thymectomy and open thymectomy: outcome analysis of 263 patients. Ann Thorac Surg 2012;94(3):974–81 [discussion: 981–2].

43. Whitson BA, Andrade RS, Mitiek MO, et al. Thoracoscopic thymectomy: technical pearls to a 21st century approach. J Thorac Dis 2013;5(2): 129–34.

44. Zielinski M, Czajkowski W, Gwozdz P, et al. Resection of thymomas with use of the new minimally-invasive technique of extended thymectomy performed through the subxiphoid-right video-thoracoscopic approach with double elevation of the sternum. Eur J Cardiothorac Surg 2013;44(2):e113–9 [discussion: e119].

Surgical Decision Making
Thymoma and Myasthenia Gravis

Giovanni M. Comacchio, MD[a,1], Giuseppe Marulli, MD, PhD[b], Marco Mammana, MD[a,1], Giuseppe Natale, MD[a,1], Marco Schiavon, MD, PhD[a,1], Federico Rea, MD[a,*]

KEYWORDS

• Thymus • Mediastinum • Myasthenia gravis • Thymoma • Surgery

KEY POINTS

- Patients with thymomatous myasthenia gravis show particular characteristics compared with patients with nonthymomatous myasthenia or patients with thymoma without myasthenia.
- The presence of thymoma in myasthenic patients should be carefully evaluated because it influences surgical management.
- Minimally invasive techniques are indicated in patients with myasthenia gravis associated with early stage thymoma.
- Surgical and anesthesia planning for advanced resections must consider possible postoperative complications related to myasthenia, particularly respiratory impairment.
- A multidisciplinary approach is fundamental to ensure the best clinical management of the myasthenic patients and to achieve complete resection in advanced stages.

INTRODUCTION

Thymic tumors are among the rarest human neoplasms, representing less of 1% of all adult cancers. Among these, thymomas represent the most frequent tumor subtype, with a yearly incidence rate of 1 to 5 per million people. Thymomas occur at almost all ages (range, 7–89 years) with a peak incidence between 55 and 65 years and with no pronounced sex predilection.[1,2]

Surgery represents the main therapeutic option, particularly in early stages, whereas in advanced stage disease a multidisciplinary approach with various combinations of chemotherapy and radiotherapy is the preferred therapeutic option. The main prognostic factors are represented by stage, World Health Organization histologic classification, and completeness of surgical resection.[3]

From a clinical point of view, patients may be asymptomatic or may exhibit local symptoms (pain, superior vena cava syndrome, respiratory insufficiency, tachycardia) related to the tumor dimension and invasion of adjacent organs, as well as systemic symptoms (fever, weight loss). In addition, thymomas can cause a great variety of autoimmune diseases.[1]

THYMOMA AND MYASTHENIA GRAVIS

Myasthenia gravis (MG) affects about 30% to 40% of patients with thymoma and represents the most common paraneoplastic syndrome. In contrast, in patients with MG a thymoma is found in 8.5% to 15% of cases, also as unexpected pathologic finding.[1,2,4] Patients with thymoma associated with MG show some clinical differences in

Disclosure Statement: The authors have nothing to disclose.
[a] Thoracic Surgery Unit, Department of Cardiologic, Thoracic and Vascular Sciences, University Hospital, Padova, Italy; [b] Thoracic Surgery Unit, Department of Emergency and Organ Transplantation, University Hospital, Bari, Italy
[1] Present address: Via Giustiniani, 2, Padova 35100, Italy.
* Corresponding author. Via Giustiniani, 2, Padova 35100, Italy.
E-mail address: federico.rea@unipd.it

comparison with those without MG. Patient with thymomatous MG are generally 10 years younger than those with thymoma without MG. Moreover, Chinese myasthenic patients have a 2- to 3-fold increased risk of developing thymoma compared with Japanese and Caucasians, showing concurrently a generally milder MG and lower anti–acetylcholine receptor antibody titers.[4–6]

Generally, the most common histotypes of thymoma are AB and B2. Types B2 and B3 tumors are more frequently associated with MG, whereas type A tumors are seldom associated with MG and, in contrast, exhibit frequent association with other paraneoplastic manifestations as hypogammaglobulinaemia.[1,7,8] This different distribution among the histologic subtypes may be explained with the observation that cortical thymomas, sharing some morphologic characteristics with the normal thymic cortex, may have the ability to stimulate the maturation of naive CD4 T cells. In this phase of maturation, epithelial neoplastic cells may express epitopes that cross-react with skeletal muscle proteins, such as acetylcholine receptor, activating the autoimmune response.[9]

Regarding the influence of MG on thymoma survival, there have been different results reported in the literature. Although earlier studies identified MG as a negative prognostic factor for long-term survival, mainly related to a suboptimal MG therapy or because its relationship with more aggressive histotypes, recent studies showed no relationship or even a prolonged overall and disease-free survival in patients with MG.[4,7,8,10] This finding may be also explained by an earlier thymoma diagnosis in patients with MG and, thus, an earlier thymectomy.[7]

Concurrently, MG in patients with thymoma seems to benefit less from thymectomy compared with nonthymomatous ones. Complete remission is described in 10% to 20% of cases after 5 years, compared with 30% to 60% in case of nonthymomatous MG; thus, thymoma is a poor prognostic factor because of the lesser response to treatment and greater severity of symptoms.[7,11–14]

CLINICAL EVALUATION

There are 2 main scenarios that the surgeon may find himself to deal with:

- Patient referred to the surgeon for a mediastinal lesion; and
- Patient referred to the surgeon for MG.

In the first case, a thorough evaluation of the patient's medical history must be performed, together with a meticulous physical examination to find fluctuating muscle weakness or any other signs or symptoms of MG. Indeed, also if there are only slight symptoms, these may not have an implication for the surgical decision making, but may influence the anesthesiologic management of the patient. Rare cases of latent MG with positive antibody titer have been described and were characterized by a protracted nondepolarizing neuromuscular blocking effect in the postoperative course.[13]

A diagnosis of MG is established through the detection of serum antibodies and may be confirmed by electromyography studies or clinical response to acetylcholinesterase inhibitors.[14] In any case, neurologic assessment is mandatory to confirm the diagnosis and establish appropriate medical therapy. Particularly, the presence of serum antibodies should be investigated in all patients with thymoma because these patients are at risk of developing postthymectomy MG. The risk of developing MG after thymectomy is about 1% to 3%; the major risk factor is a positive preoperative anti–acetylcholine receptor antibody level.[4]

In other cases, the patient is referred to the surgeon directly with a diagnosis of MG. If not already performed, the clinical evaluation should be completed with a contrast-enhanced chest computed tomography (CT) scan to evaluate the thymic region and particularly to distinguish between thymic hyperplasia and early stage thymoma. Indeed, the presence of a thymoma is an absolute indication for thymectomy, irrespective of the presence or degree of MG, whereas in case of hyperplasia the decision is based on the neurologic disease. Moreover, a CT scan is used to assess the invasion of adjacent structures and to better show small pleural/pericardial implants. Thymoma occurs as oval or round-shaped mass with mild or moderate contrast enhancement. Frequently, calcifications are detected and degenerative changes or signs of necrosis may be present.[15]

However, although chest CT is considered the routine modality in the imaging of thymic lesions, in some cases the differentiation between hyperplasia and thymoma may be ambiguous.[16] Indeed, the rate of unnecessary thymectomies carried out according only to a CT diagnosis is 43.8% (of which 17.1% are thymic hyperplasia cases).[17]

In these cases, MRI, although not routinely used in the assessment of patients with MG, may be useful to distinguish normal and hyperplastic thymus from thymic tumors. In particular, it is able to detect any fatty tissue within the normal or hyperplastic thymus, showing a homogenous signal decrease on opposed-phase chemical shift, whereas this signal loss is absent in thymic tumors that do not contain fat.[16,18] Moreover, the high contrast resolution may be useful for defining the invasion of contiguous structures and when the distinction between a cystic thymoma and a congenital thymic cyst should be made, by identification of fibrous septa or mural nodules on T2-weighted MRI.[19]

PET-CT scans with 18F-fluorodeoxyglucose (FDG) are becoming fundamental for the clinical staging of thymic tumors, particularly for the identification of nodal or distant metastases, thus guiding the therapeutic approach. However, in the diagnosis of small thymic lesions and in the differential diagnosis between thymoma and thymic hyperplasia, particularly in young patients, it has a decreased specificity. Indeed, thymoma may have very low FDG avidity, whereas normal and hyperplastic thymic tissue may be avid on 18F-FDG PET-CT scans.[18,19] Some authors evaluated the relationship between metabolic parameters of PET-CT scans and the World Health Organization histologic classification of thymic tumors and showed a significant difference in the maximum standardized uptake value parameter between low-grade (A, AB, B1) and high-grade (B2, B3) thymomas and thymic carcinoma.[15]

More invasive diagnostic approaches, such as biopsy of the, lesion may not be necessary in case of small or medium-size lesions diagnosed on imaging and without evidence of local invasion and may be resected directly. Instead, a tissue diagnosis may be necessary in case of larger lesions and to differentiate between a thymoma and a thymic carcinoma or other mediastinal tumors or in the need for induction chemotherapy.[3]

PREOPERATIVE EVALUATION

Anesthesiologic assessment of patients with thymomatous MG is similar to that for patients with MG but without thymoma. Coexisting disease should be investigated carefully, particularly those that could affect MG, such as thyroid diseases.[20,21] Particular details to pay attention are related to the surgical approach, the prolonged operative time, and the possible resection of the surrounding structures in case of thymoma.

Regarding the first point, particularly for advanced stages, an invasive open approach may be necessary to remove the tumor completely, whereas the possibility of minimally invasive approach is limited to early stages. Indeed, the more invasive the approach is, the more it influences the postoperative course, in terms of pulmonary function, need for medications, and pain relief. Sternotomy and thoracotomy produce a marked decrease in pulmonary function and this factor is particularly important in patients

with MG, where the disease itself causes an impairment of lung function, related to the weakness of the diaphragm and of the thoracic muscles. Therefore, these patients are especially prone to developing pulmonary complications after surgery. The etiology is multifactorial, but pain is one of the main factors, particularly for thoracotomy. Thus, an adequate pain-relieving therapeutic strategy should be in place. The most effective mode of analgesic administration seems to be a combination of systemic and local analgesics, as either continuous epidural analgesia or paravertebral extrapleural infusion.[21,22]

Moreover, surgical resection of thymomas may frequently require resection of adjacent organs, such as lung parenchyma or great vessels. In parenchymal resection, a thorough briefing between the surgeon and the anesthesiologist is mandatory to plan for the possible extension of the resection and thus the necessary functional evaluation and the most suitable postoperative management.[21] In resection of the great vessels, it is crucial that careful surgical planning allows for subsequent reconstruction. With limited invasion of the vessels, a direct clamping of the vessel may be sufficient, whereas in other cases there may a need for vascular shunts or cardiopulmonary bypass.

From a neurologic point of view, elective surgery for thymomatous MG should be reserved until after a stabilization of symptoms, when possible, balancing the oncological needs.[21] Neurologic optimization is fundamental to ensure an early and safe recovery in the postoperative course and to minimize the risks of myasthenic complications. In high-risk patients with a difficult control of the symptoms in the preoperative period, more aggressive approaches, such as intravenous immunoglobulin or plasmapheresis, may be considered.[23]

Postoperative myasthenic crisis is a life-threatening condition, characterized by acute exacerbation of MG symptoms with severe muscular weakness that necessitates intubation or delayed extubation after surgery.[24] Identification of high-risk patients is then useful for the anesthesiologist to plan the postoperative course, particularly regarding the duration of intubation and admission to the intensive care unit. In the literature, some investigators have detected different factors as predictive of postoperative myasthenic crisis. Recently, Leuzzi and colleagues[25] developed a predictive score for postoperative myasthenic crisis based on the Osserman stage, the duration of myasthenic symptoms, body mass index, and the association with lung resections. As stated, pulmonary function should be evaluated carefully in patients with MG both in case of pulmonary resection, and because preoperative pulmonary function is in strict relationship with the control of the disease and may predict postoperative complications. Indeed, the ratio between the measured forced expiratory volume in 1 second and predicted forced expiratory volume in 1 second and between measured forced vital capacity and predicted forced vital capacity are significantly related to the risk of myasthenic crisis after thymectomy.[26]

SURGERY

The surgical strategy is strictly related to the disease's stage (**Box 1**); thus, thorough preoperative staging is required.

Early Stages: Masaoka Stages I and II

For early stage disease (Masaoka stages I and II), surgical resection is the mainstay of therapy. Complete surgical resection ensures optimal oncological long-term results.[3] Surgery for thymomas has been traditionally performed through median sternotomy; however, in recent years minimally invasive techniques have gained attention in this field, particularly in cases of myasthenic patients, achieving comparable results both in terms of surgical, neurologic, and oncological outcomes (**Table 1**).[27–62] Concurrently, these approaches avoid some complications of open access, such as sternal instability, wound healing impairment, wound infection, hematomas.[66–68] These complications may be particularly frequent in patients with MG where, for example, the use of steroids

---

Box 1
Principles of thymectomy in patients with thymoma and myasthenia gravis

Preoperative neurologic and serologic assessment

Elective surgery and stabilization of neurologic symptoms

Thorough preoperative oncological staging

Total thymectomy with no-touch technique

Minimally invasive approach for early stage disease (in experienced centers)

R0 resection with vascular reconstruction as needed (in experienced centers)

Phrenic sparing surgical approach (if at all possible)

Awareness of postoperative myasthenia gravis–related complications (respiratory impairment)

---

has also raised controversies, because of the supposed increased risk in wound complications after sternotomy.[69]

Indeed, different studies compared sternotomy with minimally invasive approaches, showing a decrease in blood losses, complication rate, and duration of hospital stay.[38,40,46,54,56,70,71] Particularly, a better preservation of the pulmonary function is described and this issue may be fundamental for myasthenic patients, to avoid postoperative respiratory complications.[22] The lesser morbidity of minimally invasive techniques has led to a greater acceptance of these operations, especially for benign hyperplastic thymus with earlier referral of myasthenic patients to the surgeon.

From an oncological point of view, there has been a certain degree of skepticism in the early years regarding the use of minimally invasive thymectomy[72]; however, several investigators published their experiences with promising results (see **Table 1**) and a recent review and metaanalysis of the literature by Friedant and colleagues[73] showed comparable results when comparing transternal thymectomy with a minimally invasive one. To date, no published series have reached the necessary long-term duration of follow-up for thymoma to make definite conclusions; however, the results are encouraging. Because of the comparable oncological results and the decreased incidence of complications, it is now generally accepted that surgery for early stage thymomas can be safely performed with minimally invasive approaches, particularly in case of patients with MG. Referring specifically to minimally invasive techniques, there is great debate over whether one technique is superior to the others. The most widespread techniques are cervicotomy, VATS, and robotic thymectomy.

Cervicotomy represents a common approach in many centers for patients with MG or small thymomas.[74,75] However, although showing different advantages in terms of fewer postoperative complications, particularly regarding the pulmonary function and length of hospital stay, dissection of all the mediastinal fat through the single cervical incision may be challenging and frequently an additional thoracoscopic incision or a partial sternotomy is necessary.[76] Moreover, thymomas removed through cervicotomy are generally of small dimensions or incidental findings in patients with MG; thus, no clear data are available in the literature regarding the oncological outcome.

The main debate is between robotic and thoracoscopic thymectomy. Advantages of the former technique are the high-resolution 3-dimensional view and the improved dexterity of the robotic

Table 1
Major series of minimally invasive thymectomy for thymoma and MG

Author	No. of Patients	Surgical Approach	Thymoma/Nonthymoma	MG	OC (%)	Morbidity (%)	POS (d)	FU (mo)	RR (%)	Thymoma 5-y Survival (%)	MG Remission (%)
Roviaro et al,[27] 2000	22	uVATS	22/0	—	4.5	—	6[a]	—	4.5	—	—
Mineo et al,[28] 2000	31	uVATS	4/27	31	3.2	—	5.2[a]	39.6[a]	—	—	36 CSR / 96 I
Tomulescu et al,[29] 2006	107	uVATS	0/107	107	0	9.34	2.3[a]	36.4[a]	—	—	59.6 CSR
Rea et al,[30] 2006	33	Robotic	2/31	33	0	6.0	2.6[b]	28.8[a]	0	—	16.6 CSR
Cheng et al,[31] 2007	44	uVATS	44/0	15	0	0	7.6[a]	36.4[a]	0	100	—
Augustin et al,[32] 2008	32	Robotic	6/26	NA	3.1	6.2	6.0[b]	25.0[a]	0	—	—
Rückert et al,[33] 2008	95	Robotic	12/83	95	8.3	2.1	—	29.1[b]	0	—	>40 CSR
Fleck et al,[34] 2009	18	Robotic	0/18	18	5.5	33.3	4.2[a]	18.0[b]	—	—	55.5
Odaka et al,[35] 2010	22	uVATS	22/0	0	0	0	4.6[a]	21.6[a]	0	—	—
Agasthian & Lin,[36] 2010	119	uVATS	58/61	93	0	10	5.0[a]	58.8[a]	3.4	100	21
Goldstein et al,[37] 2010	26	Robotic	5/21	26	15.3	15.3	2.0[a]	26.0[a]	—	—	38.0 PR
Pennathur et al,[38] 2011	18	bVATS	18/0	7	0	—	3.0[b]	27[b]	0	100	—
Takeo et al,[39] 2011	35	bVATS	35/0	2	0	8.5	10.5[a]	65[a]	2.8	100	—
Balduyck et al,[40] 2011	14	Robotic	5/9	5	7.1	21.4	9.6[a]	34.2[a]	—	—	—
Freeman et al,[41] 2011	75	Robotic	0/75	75	0	6.6	2.2[a]	45.0[a]	—	—	53.3
Rückert et al,[42] 2011	153	Robotic[63] uVATS[64]	11/63 6/73	153	1.4 1.3	2.7 2.5	—	42.0[a]	—	—	39.3 CSR / 20.3 CSR
Mussi et al,[43] 2012	14	Robotic	14/0	1	7.7	14.2	4.0[a]	14.5[b]	0	100	100 I
Melfi et al,[44] 2012	39	Robotic	13/26	20	5.1	12.8	4.3[a]	16.0[b]	0	—	90.0 I

(continued on next page)

Table 1
(continued)

Author	No. of Patients	Surgical Approach	Thymoma/Nonthymoma	MG	OC (%)	Morbidity (%)	POS (d)	FU (mo)	RR (%)	Thymoma 5-y Survival (%)	MG Remission (%)
Marulli et al,[45] 2012	79	Robotic	79/0	45	1.3	12.7	4.4a	51.7a	1.3	97	—
Weksler et al,[46] 2012	15	Robotic	10/5	5	0	6.6	1.0b	—	—	—	—
Jurado et al,[47] 2012	77	uVATS[65] Robotic[2]	10/67	43	—	9.0	3.0b	24.2b	0	—	70 CSR
Kimura et al,[48] 2013	45	uVATS	45/0	14	0	—	11.0a	—	6.7	100	—
Marulli et al,[49] 2013	100	Robotic	8/92	100	0	6.0	3.0b	67.0b	0	100	28.5 CSR 87.5 I
Schneiter et al,[50] 2013	20	Robotic	20/0	12	0	10.0	5.0b	26.0b	11.1	100	—
Liu et al,[51] 2014	76	uVATS	76/0	35	1.3	—	7.1a	61.9a	2.6	100	—
Ye et al,[52] 2014	125	uVATS	125/0	0	3.2	4.8	8b	41.0a	0.8	—	—
Sakamaki et al,[53] 2014	71	uVATS	71/0	26	5.6	—	—	48.0b	1.4	97	73 I
Ye et al,[54] 2014	23	Robotic	23/0	0	0	4.3	3.7a	16.9a	0	100	—
Keijzers et al,[55] 2014	37	Robotic	37/0	28	13.5	16.2	3.0b	36.0b	2.7	100	21.4
Seong et al,[56] 2014	34	Robotic	11/23	2	—	0	2.7a	13.3a	0	—	—
Jun et al,[57] 2014	55	Robotic	21/34	NA	0	10.9	7.2a	—	—	—	—
Huang et al,[58] 2014	23	Robotic	23/0	1	0	4.3	3.6a	24.8a	0	—	100 I
Liu et al,[59] 2015	103	u/bVATS	0/103	103	0	18	6.7a	62.4b	—	—	46.6 CSR
Keijzers et al,[60] 2015	125	Robotic	31/94	125	4	7.2	3.0b	33.0b	6.5	—	77 I
Marulli et al,[61] 2016	134	Robotic	134/0	70	8.9	17.1	4.0b	48.0a	0.7	100	—
Kumar et al,[62] 2017	71	Robotic	21/50	71	0	7.0	—	33.0b	0	—	38 CSR

Abbreviations: bVATS, biportal video-assisted thoracoscopic surgery; CSR, complete stable remission; FU, follow-up; I, improved; MG, myasthenia gravis; NA, not available; OC, open conversion; OT, operative time; POS, postoperative stay; PR, pharmacologic remission; RR, recurrence rate; uVATS, uniportal video-assisted thoracoscopic surgery.
a Mean.
b Median.

instruments with the tremor filtering system that allows a safe dissection around vulnerable structures as nerves and vessels, compared with the long thoracoscopic instruments that do not articulate and enhance the surgeon's tremor.[61,63] In contrast, the robot lacks tactile feedback and the surgeon is placed far from the patient, in a nonsterile fashion. Finally, robotic surgery is burdened by high costs.[32] However, all studies comparing the 2 techniques did not clearly favor one technique over the other from the surgical and, more important, the oncological points of view.[42,57]

Whatever the approach, there are some peculiar characteristics that must be kept in mind when dealing with thymectomy for thymoma differently from patient with only MG. First is the appropriate selection of patients for a minimally invasive approach. Indeed, the operation must be oncologically and technically safe and complete. The most common characteristics used to select candidates for minimally invasive thymoma resection have been summarized by Cheng and colleagues[31]: the location in the anterior mediastinum, the tumor encapsulation, a distinct fat plane between the tumor and vital organs, the existence of residual normal appearing thymic tissue, no mass compression effect, and unilateral tumor predominance. Apart from the previous characteristics, tumor dimension must be considered as well; ideally, it should be considered for lesions smaller than 3 cm, although in the literature the majority of studies deal with tumors around 5 cm. Removal of thymomas up to 10 cm has been described and, although greater dimensions do not represent an absolute contraindication, they could make dissection more complex and thus should be considered only in centers with highly trained surgeons. Moreover, in the patient with MG, abundant mediastinal fat may complicate the surgical procedure.

More important, and differently from operations performed only for MG, thymomas should be resected using a "no-touch" technique; thus, particular care should be taken not to grasp the lesion directly, but to use the surrounding normal thymic tissue to manipulate the specimen because of the possibility of rupturing the capsule and increasing the risk of pleural dissemination.[63] However, this technique requires a more complex and accurate dissection of the thymus, and thus has a longer learning curve; it should be performed only by experienced surgeons.[45]

Regarding the extent of resection, independent of surgical access, thymomas should be removed with the surrounding thymic tissue and mediastinal fatty tissue, 1 one phrenic nerve (PN) to the other and from the upper horns to the pericardiophrenic angles.[3] Although for thymomas without MG there is a debate as to whether thymomectomy or partial thymectomy may be sufficient for early stage disease, with thymomatous MG there is an absolute indication for total thymectomy. Maximal thymectomy should be performed also in patients with positive levels of antibodies but without clinical signs of MG, because of the increased risk of developing postthymectomy MG, as described elsewhere in this article.

Advanced Stages: Masaoka Stages III to IV

Masaoka stage III thymomas are characterized by infiltration of the surrounding structures or organs, such as the mediastinal pleura, pericardium, lung, and great vessels, thus exhibiting heterogeneous clinical and radiological presentations. In addition, stage IV disease describes a wide range of clinical scenarios, ranging from the most common presentation of pleural implants, to lymphatic and distant metastases.

Chemotherapy may be indicated in case of stage III/IVa tumors not deemed to be directly surgically resectable, with the aim of decreasing the tumor burden, facilitating surgical resection, increasing the R0 resection rate and, possibly, downstaging the tumor.[3] The indications for induction and adjuvant therapy are the same for thymomas whether or not they are associated with MG. Most therapeutic regimens are platinum based and generally well-tolerated.[77] In case of unresectable disease, definitive chemotherapy and radiotherapy are indicated.

From a surgical point of view, the principles of resection are the same as for early stage disease; thus, complete removal of the tumor, the surrounding thymic tissue and mediastinal fat, and any involved structure is indicated.[3] Resection of small tracts of pericardium or limited lung resections are easily performed in many centers and in some cases also with minimally invasive techniques. However, more extended resection and reconstruction of vital organs, such as the superior vena cava, aorta, chest wall, and trachea, should be performed only in high-volume centers to ensure a multidisciplinary approach and experience to deal with complex cases, thus increasing the chances of a complete removal of the tumor.[3]

Among stage III disease, different studies show a worse prognosis in patients with vascular involvement, mainly related to a lower rate of complete resection because of the complex surgical procedure, and a consequently higher rate of local and distant recurrence.[78,79] Regarding myasthenic patients, the main problems to be aware of are related to possible impaired pulmonary function after surgery. This symptom may be associated to a direct resection of the pulmonary parenchyma, as previously mentioned, or to involvement of the PN.

Respiratory function impairment is common in myasthenic patients and one of the causes may be detected in the diaphragmatic weakness related to decrement in the amplitude of diaphragm muscle action potential. At the same time, PN involvement is a common issue in thymoma surgery, particularly because it has been shown to be involved in 7% to 33% of advanced thymomas.[64,80] There may be 2 eventualities: a clinical and radiological suspicion of nerve involvement before surgery or an intraoperative finding of phrenic involvement.

In cases of preoperative detection of a unilateral PN palsy, paradoxically the functional assessment is easier because the patient has already developed respiratory function impairment. Moreover, the slow development of these cases may decrease respiratory distress by means of compensatory mechanisms. Finally, the resection of the PN will not be a surgical problem and an eventual diaphragmatic plication may be considered during the operation.[81]

In case of an unexpected intraoperative finding, the decision to resect the PN in a myasthenic patient or to spare it and thus perform an incomplete resection remains challenging. In a recent study by Hamdi and colleagues,[82] no differences in disease-free and overall survival were seen in patients with or without sparing of the PN for thymoma, although there was a higher risk of recurrence in the former group. However, also in patients with spared PN, a 5% permanent postoperative diaphragmatic palsy has been described, whereas in the resected group 15% of the resected PN were not involved histologically. Possible landmarks to guide the decision may be the severity of myasthenic symptoms, the presence of comorbidities, and preoperative pulmonary function tests. Moreover, if the PN has been resected, diaphragmatic plication must be considered.[81] If the thymic tumor infiltrates both PNs, it is mandatory to spare one of them to decrease respiratory functional impairment. In cases where there is a high suspicion of bilateral involvement, minimally invasive evaluation of the nerves could be performed before deciding to perform the tumor resection by an open approach, to decrease the risks of unnecessary explorative operations.

However, these cases should be discussed within a multidisciplinary oncological team to evaluate each case individually, particularly regarding the need for adjuvant radiotherapy in patients with a spared PN, but where there may be doubts on the safety margins.

Regarding pulmonary resection, particular attention should be paid in cases of pneumonectomy. Fabre and colleagues[83] described the largest series of extrapleural pneumonectomy for Masaoka IVa thymomas in myasthenic patients (29% of all patients) showing that MG is an important risk factor for bronchopleural fistulas owing to high intake of steroids. Thus, this type of operation should be proposed cautiously to myasthenic patients or avoided if possible, opting instead for minor resections. In case of pneumonectomy, every effort should be made to wean patients from steroids, and coverage of the bronchial stump is recommended.[84]

SUMMARY

MG in patients with thymoma shows peculiar characteristics compared with nonthymomatous MG and, concurrently, there are differences with patients with thymoma without MG, probably related to different pathologic mechanisms. Surgery is the mainstay in the treatment of thymoma; thus, a precise diagnosis and staging is required to plan the most appropriate treatment. In early stage disease, complete resection of the thymus and of the tumor, particularly through minimally invasive techniques, achieves optimal results from the neurologic and oncological point of view. Particular attention must be paid to patients with MG when dealing with advanced stage thymoma with need of complex resections, particularly when involving the pulmonary parenchyma, the PNs, and the great vessels. In these cases, a multidisciplinary approach in high-volume centers allows for the achievement of the best results.

REFERENCES

1. Marx A, Ströbel P, Zettl A, et al. Thymomas. In: Travis WD, Brambilla E, Müller-Hermelink HK, et al, editors. Pathology and genetics of tumours of the lung, pleura, thymus and heart. Lyon (France): IARC press; 2004. p. 152–3.
2. Detterbeck F, Parsons A. Thymic tumors. Ann Thorac Surg 2004;77:1860e9.
3. Detterbeck F, Zeeshan A. Thymoma: current diagnosis and treatment. Chin Med J (Engl) 2013;126: 2186–91.
4. Zielinski M. Management of myasthenic patients with thymoma. Thorac Surg Clin 2011;21:47–57.
5. Teoh R, McGuire L, Wong K, et al. Increased incidence of thymoma in Chinese myasthenia gravis: possible relationship with Epstein-Barr virus. Acta Neurol Scand 1989;80:221e5.

6. Kondo K, Monden Y. Thymoma and myasthenia gravis: a clinical study of 1,089 patients from Japan. Ann Thorac Surg 2005;79:219e24.

7. Vachlas K, Zisis C, Rontogianni D, et al. Thymoma and myasthenia gravis: clinical aspects and prognosis. Asian Cardiovasc Thorac Ann 2012; 20:48–52.

8. Filosso PL, Evangelista A, Ruffini E, et al. Does myasthenia gravis influence overall survival and cumulative incidence of recurrence in thymoma patients? A Retrospective clinicopathological multicentre analysis on 797 patients. Lung Cancer 2015;88:338–43.

9. Beydoun SR, Gong H, Ashikian N, et al. Myasthenia gravis associated with invasive malignant thymoma: two case reports and a review of the literature. J Med Case Rep 2014;8:340.

10. Margaritora S, Cesario A, Cusumano G, et al. Thirty-five-year follow-up analysis of clinical and pathologic outcomes of thymoma surgery. Ann Thorac Surg 2010;89:245–52.

11. Maggi G, Casadio C, Cavallo R, et al. Thymectomy in myasthenia gravis. Results of 662 cases operated upon in 15 years. Eur J Cardiothorac Surg 1989;3: 504e11.

12. Lucchi M, Ricciardi R, Melfi F, et al. Association of thymoma and myasthenia gravis: oncological and neurological results of the surgical treatment. Eur J Cardiothorac Surg 2009;35:812–6.

13. Ito S, Fujita Y, Sasano H, et al. Latent myasthenia gravis revealed by protracted postoperative effect of non-depolarizing neuromuscular blockade. J Anesth 2012;26:953–4.

14. Evoli A, Iorio R, Bartoccioni E. Overcoming challenges in the diagnosis and treatment of myasthenia gravis. Expert Rev Clin Immunol 2016;12:157–68.

15. Otsuka H. The utility of FDG-PET in the diagnosis of thymic epithelial tumors. J Med Invest 2012;59: 225–34.

16. Priola AM, Priola SM. Imaging of thymus in myasthenia gravis: from thymic hyperplasia to thymic tumor. Clin Radiol 2014;69:e230–45.

17. Ottlakan A, Borda B, Morvay Z, et al. The effect of diagnostic imaging on surgical treatment planning in diseases of the thymus. Contrast Media Mol Imaging 2017;2017:9307292.

18. McInnis MC, Flores EJ, Shepard JA, et al. Pitfalls in the imaging and interpretation of benign thymic lesions: how thymic MRI can help. AJR Am J Roentgenol 2016;206:W1–8.

19. Marom EM. Advances in thymoma imaging. J Thorac Imaging 2013;28:69–80.

20. Sungur Z, Sentürk M. Anaesthesia for thymectomy in adult and juvenile myasthenic patients. Curr Opin Anaesthesiol 2016;29:14–9.

21. Krucylak PE, Naunheim KS. Preoperative preparation and anesthetic management of patients with myasthenia gravis. Semin Thorac Cardiovasc Surg 1999;11:47–53.

22. Rückert JC, Walter M, Müller JM. Pulmonary function after thoracoscopic thymectomy versus median sternotomy for myasthenia gravis. Ann Thorac Surg 2000;70:1656–61.

23. Skeie GO, Apostolski S, Evoli A, et al. Guidelines for treatment of autoimmune neuromuscular transmission disorders. Eur J Neurol 2010;17:893–902.

24. Wu Y, Chen Y, Liu H, et al. Risk factors for developing postthymectomy myasthenic crisis in thymoma patients. J Cancer Res Ther 2015;11:C115–7.

25. Leuzzi G, Meacci E, Cusumano G, et al. Thymectomy in myasthenia gravis: proposal for a predictive score of postoperative myasthenic crisis. Eur J Cardiothorac Surg 2014;45:e76–88.

26. Choi KH, Nam TS, Lee SH, et al. Preoperative pulmonary function is strongly related to myasthenic crisis after thymectomy. Neurol India 2014;62:164–8.

27. Roviaro G, Varoli F, Nucca O, et al. Videothoracoscopic approach to primary mediastinal pathology. Chest 2000;117:1179–83.

28. Mineo TC, Pompeo E, Lerut TE, et al. Thoracoscopic thymectomy in autoimmune myasthenia: results of left-sided approach. Ann Thorac Surg 2000;69: 1537–41.

29. Tomulescu V, Ion V, Kosa A, et al. Thoracoscopic thymectomy mid-term results. Ann Thorac Surg 2006;82:1003–7.

30. Rea F, Marulli G, Bortolotti L, et al. Experience with the "da Vinci" robotic system for thymectomy in patients with myasthenia gravis: report of 33 cases. Ann Thorac Surg 2006;81:455–9.

31. Cheng YJ, Hsu JS, Kao EL. Characteristics of thymoma successfully resected by videothoracoscopic surgery. Surg Today 2007;37:192–6.

32. Augustin F, Schmid T, Sieb M, et al. Video-assisted thoracoscopic surgery versus robotic-assisted thoracoscopic surgery thymectomy. Ann Thorac Surg 2008;85:S768–71.

33. Rückert JC, Ismail M, Swierzy M, et al. Thoracoscopic thymectomy with the da Vinci robotic system for myasthenia gravis. Ann N Y Acad Sci 2008;1132: 329–35.

34. Fleck T, Fleck M, Müller M, et al. Extended videoscopic robotic thymectomy with the da Vinci telemanipulator for the treatment of myasthenia gravis: the Vienna experience. Interact Cardiovasc Thorac Surg 2009;9:784–7.

35. Odaka M, Akiba T, Yabe M, et al. Unilateral thoracoscopic subtotal thymectomy for the treatment of stage I and II thymoma. Eur J Cardiothorac Surg 2010;37:824–6.

36. Agasthian T, Lin S. Clinical outcome of video-assisted thymectomy for myasthenia gravis and thymoma. Asian Cardiovasc Thorac Ann 2010;18: 234–9.

37. Goldstein SD, Yang SC. Assessment of robotic thymectomy using the Myasthenia Gravis Foundation of America guidelines. Ann Thorac Surg 2010;89: 1080–5.

38. Pennathur A, Qureshi I, Schuchert MJ, et al. Comparison of surgical techniques for early-stage thymoma: feasibility of minimally invasive thymectomy and comparison with open resection. J Thorac Cardiovasc Surg 2011;141:694–701.

39. Takeo S, Tsukamoto S, Kawano D, et al. Outcome of an original video-assisted thoracoscopic extended thymectomy for thymoma. Ann Thorac Surg 2011; 92:2000–5.

40. Balduyck B, Hendriks JM, Lauwers P, et al. Quality of life after anterior mediastinal mass resection: a prospective study comparing open with robotic-assisted thoracoscopic resection. Eur J Cardiothorac Surg 2011;39:543–8.

41. Freeman RK, Ascioti AJ, Van Woerkom JM, et al. Long-term follow-up after robotic thymectomy for nonthymomatous myasthenia gravis. Ann Thorac Surg 2011;92:1018–22.

42. Rückert JC, Swierzy M, Ismail M. Comparison of robotic and nonrobotic thoracoscopic thymectomy: a cohort study. J Thorac Cardiovasc Surg 2011;141: 673–7.

43. Mussi A, Fanucchi O, Davini F, et al. Robotic extended thymectomy for early-stage thymomas. Eur J Cardiothorac Surg 2012;41:e43–6.

44. Melfi F, Fanucchi O, Davini F, et al. Ten-year experience of mediastinal robotic surgery in a single referral centre. Eur J Cardiothorac Surg 2012;41: 847–51.

45. Marulli G, Rea F, Melfi F, et al. Robot-aided thoracoscopic thymectomy for early-stage thymoma: a multicenter European study. J Thorac Cardiovasc Surg 2012;144:1125–30.

46. Weksler B, Tavares J, Newhook TE, et al. Robot-assisted thymectomy is superior to transsternal thymectomy. Surg Endosc 2012;26:261–6.

47. Jurado J, Javidfar J, Newmark A, et al. Minimally invasive thymectomy and open thymectomy: outcome analysis of 263 patients. Ann Thorac Surg 2012;94:974–81.

48. Kimura T, Inoue M, Kadota Y, et al. The oncological feasibility and limitations of video-assisted thoracoscopic thymectomy for early-stage thymomas. Eur J Cardiothorac Surg 2013;44:e214–8.

49. Marulli G, Schiavon M, Perissinotto E, et al. Surgical and neurologic outcomes after robotic thymectomy in 100 consecutive patients with myasthenia gravis. J Thorac Cardiovasc Surg 2013;145:730–5.

50. Schneiter D, Tomaszek S, Kestenholz P, et al. Minimally invasive resection of thymomas with the da Vinci® Surgical System. Eur J Cardiothorac Surg 2013;43:288–92.

51. Liu TJ, Lin MW, Hsieh MS, et al. Video-assisted thoracoscopic surgical thymectomy to treat early thymoma: a comparison with the conventional transsternal approach. Ann Surg Oncol 2014;21: 322–8.

52. Ye B, Tantai JC, Ge XX, et al. Surgical techniques for early-stage thymoma: video-assisted thoracoscopic thymectomy versus transsternal thymectomy. J Thorac Cardiovasc Surg 2014;147:1599–603.

53. Sakamaki Y, Oda T, Kanazawa G, et al. Intermediate-term oncologic outcomes after video-assisted thoracoscopic thymectomy for early-stage thymoma. J Thorac Cardiovasc Surg 2014;148:1230–7.

54. Ye B, Li W, Ge XX, et al. Surgical treatment of early-stage thymomas: robot-assisted thoracoscopic surgery versus transsternal thymectomy. Surg Endosc 2014;28:122–6.

55. Keijzers M, Dingemans AM, Blaauwgeers H, et al. 8 years' experience with robotic thymectomy for thymomas. Surg Endosc 2014;28:1202–8.

56. Seong YW, Kang CH, Choi JW, et al. Early clinical outcomes of robot-assisted surgery for anterior mediastinal mass: its superiority over a conventional sternotomy approach evaluated by propensity score matching. Eur J Cardiothorac Surg 2014;45:e68–73.

57. Jun Y, Hao L, Demin L, et al. Da Vinci robot-assisted system for thymectomy: experience of 55 patients in China. Int J Med Robot 2014;10:294–9.

58. Huang P, Ye B, Yang Y, et al. Experience with the "da Vinci" robotic system for early-stage thymomas: report of 23 cases. Thorac Cancer 2014;5:325–9.

59. Liu Z, Yang J, Lin L, et al. Unilateral video-assisted thoracoscopic extended thymectomy offers long-term outcomes equivalent to that of the bilateral approach in the treatment of non-thymomatous myasthenia gravis. Interact Cardiovasc Thorac Surg 2015;21:610–5.

60. Keijzers M, de Baets M, Hochstenbag M, et al. Robotic thymectomy in patients with myasthenia gravis: neurological and surgical outcomes. Eur J Cardiothorac Surg 2015;48:40–5.

61. Marulli G, Maessen J, Melfi F, et al. Multi-institutional European experience of robotic thymectomy for thymoma. Ann Cardiothorac Surg 2016;5:18–25.

62. Kumar A, Goyal V, Asaf BB, et al. Robotic thymectomy for myasthenia gravis with or without thymoma-surgical and neurological outcomes. Neurol India 2017;65:58–63.

63. Ismail M, Swierzy M, Rückert JC. State of the art of robotic thymectomy. World J Surg 2013;37:2740–6.

64. Salati M, Cardillo G, Carbone L, et al. Iatrogenic phrenic nerve injury during thymectomy: the extent of the problem. J Thorac Cardiovasc Surg 2010; 139:e77–8.

65. Toker A, Sonett J, Zielinski M, et al. Standard terms, definitions, and policies for minimally invasive resection of thymoma. J Thorac Oncol 2011;6:S1739–42.

66. Chetta A, Bobbio A, Aiello M, et al. Changes in lung function and respiratory muscle strength after sternotomy vs. laparotomy in patients without ventilatory limitation. Eur Surg Res 2006;38:489–93.

67. Kalso E, Mennander S, Tasmuth T, et al. Chronic post-sternotomy pain. Acta Anaesthesiol Scand 2001;45:935–9.

68. Marulli G, Comacchio GM, Stocca F, et al. Robotic-assisted thymectomy: current perspectives. Robotic Surg Res Rev 2016;3:53–63.

69. Zieliński M, Kuzdzał J, Staniec B, et al. Safety for preoperative use of steroids for transsternal thymectomy in myasthenia gravis. Eur J Cardiothorac Surg 2004;26:407–11.

70. Cheng YJ, Kao EL, Chou SH. Videothoracoscopic resection of stage II thymoma: prospective comparison of the results between thoracoscopy and open methods. Chest 2005;128:3010–2.

71. Cakar F, Werner P, Augustin F, et al. A comparison of outcomes after robotic open extended thymectomy for myasthenia gravis. Eur J Cardiothorac Surg 2007;31:501–4.

72. Davenport E, Malthaner RA. The role of surgery in the management of thymoma: a systematic review. Ann Thorac Surg 2008;86:673–84.

73. Friedant AJ, Handorf EA, Su S, et al. Minimally invasive versus open thymectomy for thymic malignancies: systematic review and meta-analysis. J Thorac Oncol 2016;11:30–8.

74. Maggi G, Giaccone G, Donadio M, et al. Thymomas. A review of 169 cases, with particular reference to results of surgical treatment. Cancer 1986;58: 765–76.

75. de Perrot M, Bril V, McRae K, et al. Impact of minimally invasive trans-cervical thymectomy on outcome in patients with myasthenia gravis. Eur J Cardiothorac Surg 2003;24:677–83.

76. Shrager JB, Nathan D, Brinster CJ, et al. Outcomes after 151 extended transcervical thymectomies for myasthenia gravis. Ann Thorac Surg 2006;82: 1863–9.

77. Rea F, Sartori F, Loy M, et al. Chemotherapy and operation for invasive thymoma. J Thorac Cardiovasc Surg 1993;106:543–9.

78. Marulli G, Lucchi M, Margaritora S, et al. Surgical treatment of stage III thymic tumors: a multi-institutional review from four Italian centers. Eur J Cardiothorac Surg 2011;39:e1–7.

79. Okumura M, Miyoshi S, Takeuchi Y, et al. Results of surgical treatment of thymomas with special reference to the involved organs. J Thorac Cardiovasc Surg 1999;117:605–13.

80. Yano M, Sasaki H, Moriyama S, et al. Preservation of phrenic nerve involved by stage III thymoma. Ann Thorac Surg 2010;89:1612–9.

81. Gaissert H, Wilcox SR. Diaphragmatic dysfunction after thoracic operations. Thorac Cardiovasc Surg 2016;64:621–30.

82. Hamdi S, Mercier O, Fadel E, et al. Is scarifying the phrenic nerve during thymoma resection worthwhile? Eur J Cardiothorac Surg 2014;45:e151–5.

83. Fabre D, Fadel E, Mussot S, et al. Long-term outcome of pleuropneumonectomy for Masaoka stage Iva thymoma. Eur J Cardiothorac Surg 2011; 39:e133–8.

84. Hamad AM, Marulli G, Sartori F, et al. Pericardial flap for bronchial stump coverage after extrapleural pneumonectomy; is it feasible? Eur J Cardiothorac Surg 2008;34:1255–6.

Non-Myasthenia Gravis Immune Syndromes and the Thymus
Is There a Role for Thymectomy?

Sean C. Wightman, MD, Joseph B. Shrager, MD*

KEYWORDS

- Immune syndrome • Autoimmune disease • Thymic epithelial tumor • Thymoma • Thymectomy

KEY POINTS

- Thymectomies are attempted for nonmyasthenic immune syndromes with varying degrees of success.
- Only case reports and a few small series document patient outcomes after thymectomies; no randomized control trials exist.
- Some immune syndromes, such as pure red cell aplasia, pemphigus, rheumatoid arthritis, autoimmune hemolytic anemia, and ulcerative colitis, warrant further pursuit.

INTRODUCTION

Thymectomy has been considered, performed, and discussed for many different immune syndromes beyond myasthenia gravis (MG) over the last century. These have included thymectomies performed both with and without the presence of a thymic epithelial tumors (TET). The degree of symptom improvement after thymectomy for these non-MG syndromes has been variable.[1,2] Although numerous reports exist documenting the association of immune syndromes with TETs, few address the role thymectomy on resolution of the syndromes, and most of these are case reports of little scientific validity.[3]

Owing to the rarity of performing a thymectomy for non-MG immune syndromes, little consensus on indications exist. Immune syndromes associated with TETs include pure red cell aplasia, pemphigus, peripheral nerve hyperexcitability syndromes, Good syndrome, lichen planus, Graves disease, Sjögren syndrome, and scleroderma. Immune syndromes for which thymectomy has been

performed only in patients without an associated indication to resect a TET include rheumatoid arthritis (RA), multiple sclerosis (MS), and Crohn disease. Inflammatory myopathies, autoimmune hemolytic anemia (AIHA), systemic lupus erythematosus (SLE), immune thrombocytopenia (ITP), and ulcerative colitis (UC) are immune syndromes for which thymectomy has been attempted for patients both with and without an associated TET.

For this review, we sought to identify all case reports and series in the literature relevant to this topic. An attempt was made to summarize the case reports and patients' responses to thymectomy. We grouped the responses into four categories; remission (no additional therapy/ symptoms), improvement (less therapy/symptoms), no change (same therapy/symptoms), and worsening (increased therapy/symptoms).

Because none of these series or cases are randomized, patients vary in terms of disease severity and associated treatments, including immunosuppressive medications. There may be a large degree of publication bias present favoring only successful

Disclosure Statement: The authors have nothing to disclose.
Division of Thoracic Surgery, Department of Cardiothoracic Surgery, Stanford University Hospitals and Clinics, 300 Pasteur Drive, Stanford, CA 94305, USA
* Corresponding author.
E-mail address: shrager@stanford.edu

case reports. On the other hand, most attempts at thymectomy in immune syndromes occurred after a patient was refractory to other treatments, and thus these patients typically have a more severe manifestation of their immune syndrome.

It is our belief that, as for MG, thymectomy for non-MG immune syndromes requires the surgeon to perform at least an "extended thymectomy," with removal of the entire intracapsular thymus gland as well as all fatty and thymic tissue between the phrenic nerves and down to the level of the diaphragm. We consider that this can be achieved by a variety of surgical approaches, including the transcervical approach (in the absence of a TET), which is favored by our group[4] and is now performed by us with video-thoracoscopic assistance.[5]

THYMECTOMY FOR NON-MYASTHENIA GRAVIS IMMUNE SYNDROMES WITH ASSOCIATED THYMIC EPITHELIAL TUMORS

TETs vary in aggressiveness from indolent to invasive malignancy. There are 3 existing theories of why TETs are associated with immune syndromes, reviewed by Bernard and colleagues.[6] Only case reports and small case series exist in the literature describing response to thymectomy for non-MG immune syndromes that are associated with TETs. The immune syndromes highlighted here include pure red cell aplasia, pemphigus, peripheral nerve hyperexcitability syndromes, Good syndrome, lichen planus, Graves disease, Sjögren syndrome, and scleroderma.

Pure Red Cell Aplasia

Pure red cell aplasia (PRCA) is an autoimmune cytopenia with the absence of reticulocytes in the blood and absence of erythroid precursors in the bone marrow.[6] PRCA is associated with large-cell granular lymphocyte leukemia, TETs, solid tumors, SLE, and viral infections, and is found in 5% to 10% of patients with a TET.[7,8] Apart from MG, PRCA is the immune syndrome for which thymectomy has been most aggressively pursued in the last decade.

Three case series have been published on PRCA and thymectomy. Masaoka and colleagues[9] reported 6 patients who improved but required additional therapy after thymectomy. Thompson and Steensma[10] reported 12 patients who underwent thymectomy. Although confounded by 4 patients who developed PRCA after thymectomy, 4 improved with medical therapy and 8 required regular transfusions.[10] A third series of 5 patients reported no remissions after thymectomy, although 60% improved.[11]

Overall, 46 PRCA patients who underwent thymectomy are reported in the literature, all associated with a TET. After thymectomy, remission occurred in 19 cases (41%)[8,12–26] and improvement in 18 (39%).[9,11,27–34] Symptoms were unchanged in 7 cases (16%)[35–41] and worsened in 2 (4%).[13,14] Our case compilation demonstrates a higher remission rate in refractory PRCA than previously reported in the literature.[25,42] Because a high percentage of those with refractory PRCA had remission or improved, the data are relatively convincing that thymectomy for a TET in a patient with PRCA will undergo improvement.

Pemphigus

Pemphigus is an immune syndrome that causes blistering of the skin as cell-to-cell adhesion is lost as a result of autoantibodies targeting desmoglein.[7,43] Pemphigus is associated with TET but also with other malignancies.[6] A review of thymectomy for pemphigus in the Japanese literature by Takeshita and colleagues[44] revealed 5 patients with pemphigus and a TET, and these are included in our cumulative analysis. Overall, after thymectomy remission occurred in 1 case (7%)[45] and improvement in 8 (58%).[44,46–52] Symptoms were unchanged in 3 cases (21%)[53–55] and worsened in 2 (14%).[56,57] These data suggest improvement in pemphigus symptoms after thymectomy, but most patients also required ongoing medical therapy to keep the disease under control. For pemphigus it does seem likely that thymectomy, at least with a coexisting TET, may improve the disease.

Peripheral Nerve Hyperexcitability Syndromes

Peripheral nerve hyperexcitability is a broad diagnosis that includes Isaacs and Morvan syndromes. The differences between the syndromes in this category depend on symptoms and electromyography criteria. Patients with both diseases have anti–voltage-gated potassium channel-complex antibodies in their serum. Symptoms of Isaacs syndrome include myokymia, fasciculations, muscle cramps, and hyperhidrosis.[58] Twenty percent of patients with Isaacs syndrome have an associated TET.[6] Only 6 cases of Isaacs syndrome and thymectomy for a TET are reported. Symptom remission occurred in 2 cases (33%)[6,59] with improvement in 1 (17%).[60] Symptoms worsened in 3 cases (50%).[6,61,62]

Morvan syndrome presents with myokymia, muscle pain, central nervous system symptoms, sleep disorder, and autonomic dysfunction.[58,63] Lee and colleagues[64] reported the case of a refractory patient who underwent thymectomy. With ongoing low-dose steroids, the patient's symptoms improved. In 2012, a total of 28 cases of Morvan syndrome were reviewed and 14 of these patients (50%) had a thymoma.[63] To date, this series review is still accurate with only one additional case.[65] On review of these included cases, only 8 patients underwent thymectomy and reported symptom follow-up. Remission occurred in 1 case (12%)[63] and improvement in 3 (38%).[64,66,67] Symptoms were unchanged in 4 cases (50%).[65,68–70]

The data are thus weak regarding the benefit of thymectomy in the treatment of Isaacs or Morvan syndromes.

Good Syndrome

Good syndrome consists of a triad B cell lymphopenia, hypogammaglobulinemia, and a TET, and is frequently associated with recurrent opportunistic infections.[23,71] Many clinicians advocate for investigative testing for Good syndrome in any patient with a TET and immunodeficiency or recurrent infections.[72,73]

The current treatment recommendations consist of thymectomy for the TET and immunoglobulin replacement, although mortality approaches 50%.[6,71] Nineteen case reports have been published on patients with Good syndrome who underwent thymectomy with symptom follow-up. Improvement, usually manifesting as decreased infection, was found in 8 cases (42%)[6,23,72,74–77] and symptoms were unchanged in 11 (58%).[22,23,31,78–85] No improvement in hypogammaglobulinemia was shown, and there are no case reports wherein the postoperative immunoglobulin therapy was discontinued.[23,71,84]

Based on these data, if a patient can tolerate thymectomy it should primarily be performed as treatment of the TET associated with Good syndrome, rather than with optimism that the syndrome itself will improve.

Lichen Planus

Lichen planus is an immune syndrome whereby autoreactive T cells target keratinocytes, often of the oral mucosa.[6] A recent literature review reported 30 cases of lichen planus associated with a TET but did not comment on postoperative symptoms.[6] Only 7 cases of TET-associated lichen planus underwent thymectomy with symptom follow-up. After thymectomy, symptom remission occurred in 2 cases (29%).[86,87] Symptoms worsened in 1 (14%)[88] and were unchanged in 4 cases (57%).[89–92]

Graves Disease

Graves disease is an immune syndrome whereby autoantibodies cause increased synthesis of thyroid hormone by activating thyrotropin receptors. Symptoms include hyperthyroidism, enlargement of the thyroid gland, exophthalmos, and pretibial myxedema. Treatment options include medical therapy or thyroidectomy. Two case reports exist on patients who underwent thymectomy for TET but also had ongoing Graves disease treated medically.[3,93] In both cases, the patients were made euthyroid by thymectomy. Given that these are the only case reports for Graves disease associated with a TET, it is difficult to draw any conclusion on the role of thymectomy.

Sjögren syndrome

Sjögren syndrome (SS) is an immune syndrome whereby the glands of the body produce less fluid leading to xerostomia, keratoconjunctivitis sicca, xeroderma, and vaginal dryness. To date there are 4 reported cases of SS and associated TET.[3,94–96] Seventy-five percent of the published cases of SS treatment showed no change after thymectomy. It is thus difficult to conclude that any benefit is derived from thymectomy for SS.

Scleroderma

Scleroderma is an immune syndrome that targets collagen and alters skin, vasculature, muscles, and the gastrointestinal tract. Some symptoms include Raynaud phenomenon, gastroesophageal reflux disease, interstitial lung disease, and muscle dysfunction. One case report in the literature discussed scleroderma and an associated TET. Ben-Shahar and colleagues[97] reported no improvement after thymectomy.

Section Summary

It has been noted that survival and recurrence-free survival after thymectomy for a TET is higher in patients with concomitant immune syndromes.[98] As seen from the preceding paragraphs, the literature is variable on the success of thymectomy in non-MG immune syndromes associated with TETs, but is strongest for an effect in PRCA and pemphigus. Certainly, however, in all of these diseases treatment of the thymoma will be the driving force toward performing thymectomy, rather than treatment of the associated immune syndrome. The evidence is likely not sufficiently strong to recommend thymectomy in any of these diseases in the absence of an associated thymoma.

THYMECTOMY FOR IMMUNE SYNDROMES WITHOUT ASSOCIATED THYMIC EPITHELIAL TUMORS

Thymectomy in the absence of associated TET has been attempted in the treatment of 3 non-MG immune syndromes: RA, MS, and Crohn disease.

Rheumatoid Arthritis

Thymectomies for RA, along with symptom follow-up, are documented in 10 case reports. Milne and colleagues[99] documented 2 cases of RA in which thymectomy was performed without TET and 1 patient improved. Szobor and Molnár[100,101] published a series of 4 patients who underwent thymectomy for non–TET-associated MG with simultaneous RA, 3 of whom went into remission and 1 improved. Tellez-Zenteno and colleagues[102] also published a series of 4 patients who were undergoing thymectomy for MG but had RA; 2 of these patients demonstrated improvement and remission whereas 2 patients worsened. Overall, remission occurred in 3 cases (30%)[100–102] and improvement in 4 (40%).[99–102] Symptoms worsened in 2 case (20%)[102] and were unchanged in 1 (10%).[99] Given that 70% of patients with refractory RA had symptom remission or improvement, it seems that thymectomy for the treatment of RA is worthy of further research.

Multiple Sclerosis

MS has a complex pathogenesis with T-cell–mediated demyelination of the central nervous system.[103,104] Although there may be a minor noninflammatory subtype, most consider MS to be an autoimmune disease.[103,105] Ferguson and colleagues[106] published a 35-patient series in which 1 group had combination treatment of thymectomy and azathioprine with subsequent improvement in total function and decreased exacerbations over those undergoing thymectomy alone. Three-year follow-up did not show significant improvement, and any improvement was attributed to the immunosuppression and not the thymectomy.[107] A 29-patient series by Veĭn and colleagues[108] demonstrated that those whose course was steroid-refractory had an increased sensitivity to corticosteroids after thymectomy when compared with a steroid-only control group.[2,104] Sixty-seven percent of patients noted an improvement in symptoms, but 31% developed a relapse.[104,108] Of note, the most severe patients underwent thymectomy.[2,108] There is a paucity of data on thymectomy and MS in recent decades, and no studies comparing thymectomy with modern MS treatments have been performed. The older results do not seem sufficiently impressive to consider pursuing this today.

Crohn Disease

Crohn disease is known to be associated with other autoimmune diseases. A 21-year-old patient with concomitant Crohn disease and MG was reported.[109] Her Crohn disease was previously treated with total colectomy and ileostomy but she persisted with perineal disease. After thymectomy, her Crohn disease completely remitted. Because this is the only reported case of thymectomy in a patient with Crohn disease, the documented remission rate is 100%.

Section Summary

Of the 3 immune syndromes whereby thymectomy was attempted only in the absence of TET (ie, for nonthymomatous disease), RA may be the only disease for which sufficient anecdotal evidence may warrant further study.

THYMECTOMY FOR NON-MYASTHENIA GRAVIS IMMUNE SYNDROMES WITH AND WITHOUT ASSOCIATED THYMIC EPITHELIAL TUMORS

For a few immune syndromes, thymectomy has been attempted as treatment in patients both with and without associated TETs. These syndromes include inflammatory myopathies, AIHA, SLE, ITP, and UC.

Inflammatory Myopathies

Polymyositis and dermatomyositis represent 1% to 5% of the immune syndromes associated with TET.[6] Lane and Hudson[110] published a case of thymectomy for MG and polymyositis with symptom improvement. Szobor and Molnár[100] published a case in which both polymyositis and MG had long-term remission. These are the only cases for thymectomy in polymyositis without associated TET; 1 patient improved (50%) and 1 went into remission (50%). Seven cases exist involving patients with TETs and subsequent thymectomy. Symptom remission occurred in 3 cases (42%)[111–113] and improved in 2 (30%),[114,115] whereas symptoms were unchanged in 1 (14%)[116] and worsened in 1 (14%).[115] The results of thymectomy for polymyositis have thus shown mixed outcomes, and thymectomy should not be generally recommended.

Dermatomyositis is a type of inflammatory myopathy associated with a rash and worsening muscle weakness over time. Cumming[117] reported the use of thymectomy in refractory dermatomyositis in the absence of associated TET, after which the patient remitted. Ago and colleagues[118] discussed a patient with biopsy-proven dermatomyositis, MG, and a TET. After thymectomy, dermatomyositis and MG both went into remission, but she remained on low-dose (5 mg/d) prednisolone for unclear symptoms. These two cases represent the entirety of the literature on thymectomy for dermatomyositis, and thus demonstrate 100% remission because of its rarity.

Autoimmune Hemolytic Anemia

AIHA is an autoimmune cytopenia that occurs when antibodies target blood cells causing lysis and anemia. A recent case report and literature review conducted in 2014 reported 17 cases of patients with TET and AIHA, although not all underwent thymectomy.[119] For those cases presenting with a TET at the time of thymectomy, remission occurred in 6 (75%)[119–124] with improvement in 1 (13%).[125] Symptoms were unchanged in 1 case (13%).[27] Historically, thymectomy was attempted as treatment for those with AIHA in the absence of a TET; it was attempted in 7 cases in the literature.[126] In adults, 1 remitted (50%)[126] and 1 improved (50%).[127] For the 5 children, 3 remitted (60%)[128–130] and 2 worsened (40%).[131,132] It seems, therefore, that for refractory AIHA with or without a TET, it is not unreasonable to consider thymectomy.

Systemic Lupus Erythematosus

Thymectomy has also been attempted empirically for SLE.[2,99] A series published by Milne and colleagues[99] in 1967 revealed mixed results, whereby of the 3 patients with refractory SLE who underwent thymectomy, only 1 (33%) remitted.

For patients with a TET, incidence of SLE is 1.5% to 10%.[6,133] Boonen and colleagues[134] reviewed the SLE literature and found 11 additional cases of SLE with thymomas, but without comment on symptom follow-up. There are 22 published cases of patients with SLE and TETs with symptom follow-up. After thymectomy, symptom remission occurred in 4 of these patients (18%)[135–138] with improvement in 4 (18%).[139–142] Symptoms worsened in 6 patients (28%)[6,134,138,143,144] and were unchanged in 8 (36%).[6,54,92,138,143,145] Given these data, a consistent recommendation for thymectomy in SLE does not seem warranted.

Immune Thrombocytopenia

ITP is an autoimmune disease whereby self-antibodies target platelet surface antigen. Refractory ITP often necessitates splenectomy, although Szobor and Molnár[100,101] published a series of 2 MG patients who underwent thymectomy and had resolution of their ITP. This is clearly too few patients on which to base any recommendations.

Ulcerative Colitis

In the 1970s, an immunologic etiology was found in UC.[146] In Japan, 78 patients with refractory UC underwent thymectomy (in absence of TET).[147] Outcomes in these patients were compared with those of 11 refractory patients who declined thymectomy and continued treatment with immunosuppressive agents. Patient outcomes were measured according to the percentage of patient-months the patients were symptom free. In the thymectomy group, the symptom-free patient-months before thymectomy were 60.6% and after thymectomy improved to 84.5% at 3 years. The 11 patients who declined thymectomy had only 67.8% of their patient-months symptom free.[147] Although the sample size is small, the symptom-free patient-months remained significantly higher for those undergoing thymectomy.[147] A subset of these thymectomy patients were initially published by the same group in 1984,[146] whereby 44 patients undergoing thymectomy were symptom free in 83.9% of patient-months.

Based on this prospective trial from Japan, we have attempted to organize a prospective randomized study at our institution of the role of thymectomy in UC. However, the availability of increasingly effective nonsurgical options to treat UC has dampened interest among our gastroenterologists to date.

In addition to the Japanese Ulcerative Colitis series addressing thymectomy in the absence of TET, a case report of a woman treated with thymectomy for an invasive thymoma had resolution of her UC.[148] This places the documented remission rate for UC associated with TET at 100%.

Section Summary

For most of the aforementioned immune syndromes both with and without an associated TET for which thymectomy was used, it is difficult to make recommendations because the numbers of cases are so low. However, for UC, with a substantial "n," patients were symptom free for 85% of the months followed. If thymectomy was able to spare patients colectomy, stoma, ileal pouch–anal anastomosis, or a lifetime of immunosuppressive medication, then it might represent appropriate therapy, particularly with the availability of minimally invasive thymectomy approaches. We are thus of the opinion that a comparative trial of thymectomy versus best immunosuppressive therapy should be considered.

DISCUSSION

Although there exist a few case series and many case reports, there remains no standard of care regarding when to recommend thymectomy in the management of any non-MG immune syndromes. Thus, aside from patients who have a coexistent immune syndrome and TET, the indications for surgery are unclear. Furthermore, although there remains a strong association between immune syndromes and TETs, the relative rarity of their coexistence and the paucity of literature reporting thymectomy's effect on the immune syndrome render it difficult to know the true expectation one should have for postoperative improvement. Thymectomy should also be considered in patients with immune syndromes that are refractory to other therapies among those without a TET, although deciding when to proceed with this will always be difficult.

We believe that the data suggesting an improved course for a non-MG immune syndrome after thymectomy is strongest in the cases of PRCA, pemphigus, RA, AIHA, and UC. It would be appropriate to consider clinical trials to provide further information on a possible therapeutic role of thymectomy in these diseases.

Certainly, when thymectomy is performed for the treatment of any immune syndrome, an extended thymectomy must be performed, as is done for MG. In addition to the intracapsular thymus, including the entirety of the upper horns, all mediastinal fat should be resected from the diaphragm inferiorly to the innominate veins superiorly and to the bilateral phrenic nerves laterally.[1,149,150] If done via a minimally invasive approach, such as video-assisted transcervical thymectomy, the cost and the morbidity of this intervention would undoubtedly be very low.[1]

REFERENCES

1. Shrager JB, Deeb ME, Mick R, et al. Transcervical thymectomy for myasthenia gravis achieves results comparable to thymectomy by sternotomy. Ann Thorac Surg 2002;74(2):320–6.
2. D'Andrea V, Malinovsky L, Ambrogi V, et al. Thymectomy as treatment of autoimmune diseases other than myasthenia gravis. Thymus 1993;21(1): 1–10.
3. Levy Y, Afek A, Sherer Y, et al. Malignant thymoma associated with autoimmune diseases: a retrospective study and review of the literature. Semin Arthritis Rheum 1998;28(2):73–9.
4. Shrager JB, Nathan D, Brinster CJ, et al. Outcomes after 151 extended transcervical thymectomies for myasthenia gravis. Ann Thorac Surg 2006;82(5): 1863–9.
5. Donahoe L, Keshavjee S. Video-assisted transcervical thymectomy for myasthenia gravis. Ann Cardiothorac Surg 2015;4(6):561–3.
6. Bernard C, Frih H, Pasquet F, et al. Thymoma associated with autoimmune diseases: 85 cases and literature review. Autoimmun Rev 2016;15(1): 82–92.
7. Sherer Y, Bardayan Y, Shoenfeld Y. Thymoma, thymic hyperplasia, thymectomy and autoimmune diseases (review). Int J Oncol 1997;10(5):939–43.
8. Lucchi M, Viti A, Ricciardi R, et al. Four thymus-related syndromes in a case of invasive thymoma. J Thorac Cardiovasc Surg 2007;134(5):1376–8.
9. Masaoka A, Hashimoto T, Shibata K, et al. Thymomas associated with pure red cell aplasia. Histologic and follow-up studies. Cancer 1989;64(9): 1872–8.
10. Thompson CA, Steensma DP. Pure red cell aplasia associated with thymoma: clinical insights from a 50-year single-institution experience. Br J Haematol 2006;135(3):405–7.
11. Bhargava R, Dolai TK, Singhal D, et al. Pure red cell aplasia associated with thymoma: Is thymectomy the cure? Leuk Res 2009;33(3):e17–8.
12. Mizobuchi S, Yamashiro T, Nonami Y, et al. Pure red cell aplasia and myasthenia gravis with thymoma: a case report and review of the literature. Jpn J Clin Oncol 1998;28(11):696–701.
13. Murakawa T, Nakajima J, Sato H, et al. Thymoma associated with pure red-cell aplasia: clinical features and prognosis. Asian Cardiovasc Thorac Ann 2002;10(2):150–4.
14. Vohra LS, Talwar R, Mathur M, et al. Ectopic thymoma with pure red cell aplasia—ambiguity with indolence. Int J Surg 2008;6(6):e12–4.
15. Lin CS, Yu YB, Hsu HS, et al. Pure red cell aplasia and hypogammaglobulinemia in a patient with thymoma. J Chin Med Assoc 2009;72(1):34–8.
16. Levinson AI, Hoxie JA, Kornstein MJ, et al. Absence of the OKT4 epitope on blood T cells and thymus cells in a patient with thymoma, hypogammaglobulinemia, and red blood cell aplasia. J Allergy Clin Immunol 1985;76(3):433–9.
17. Earlywine GR, Rubio FA Jr. Pure red cell aplasia with thymoma: a case report and brief review of pathogenesis. J Fla Med Assoc 1981;68(11): 890–4.
18. Aquilina A, Camilleri DJ, Aquilina J. Pure red cell aplasia and myasthenia gravis: a patient having both autoimmune conditions in the absence of thymoma. BMJ Case Rep 2017;2017 [pii:bcr-2017-220188].
19. Khalid U, Fatimi S, Saleem T. Pure red cell aplasia regression after thymus resection. Langenbecks Arch Surg 2010;395(3):289–90.
20. al-Mondhiry H, Zanjani ED, Spivack M, et al. Pure red cell aplasia and thymoma: loss of serum inhibitor of erythropoiesis following thymectomy. Blood 1971;38(5):576–82.
21. Poullis M, Punjabi P. Concomitant thymectomy and cardiac operation in a patient with pure red cell aplasia. Ann Thorac Surg 2001;72(2):621–3.

22. van der Marel J, Pahlplatz PV, Steup WH, et al. Thymoma with paraneoplastic syndromes, Good's syndrome, and pure red cell aplasia. J Thorac Oncol 2007;2(4):325–6.

23. Miyakis S, Pefanis A, Passam FH, et al. Thymoma with immunodeficiency (Good's syndrome): review of the literature apropos three cases. Scand J Infect Dis 2006;38(4):314–9.

24. Jiang D, Wu M. Thymectomy resulted in complete remission of pure red cell aplasia when associated with thymoma. Thorac Cardiovasc Surg 2010; 58(4):235–6.

25. Koizumi K, Nakao S, Haseyama Y, et al. Severe aplastic anemia associated with thymic carcinoma and partial recovery of hematopoiesis after thymectomy. Ann Hematol 2003;82(6):367–70.

26. Ito M, Imoto S, Nakagawa T, et al. Spontaneous remission in pure red cell aplasia associated with thymoma. Int J Hematol 1991;54(3):209–12.

27. Taniguchi S, Shibuya T, Morioka E, et al. Demonstration of three distinct immunological disorders on erythropoiesis in a patient with pure red cell aplasia and autoimmune haemolytic anaemia associated with thymoma. Br J Haematol 1988; 68(4):473–7.

28. Handa SI, Schofield KP, Sivakumaran M, et al. Pure red cell aplasia associated with malignant thymoma, myasthenia gravis, polyclonal large granular lymphocytosis and clonal thymic T cell expansion. J Clin Pathol 1994;47(7):676–9.

29. Lahiri TK, Agrawal D, Agrawal K, et al. Pure red cell aplasia associated with thymoma. Indian J Chest Dis Allied Sci 2002;44(4):259–62.

30. Rosu C, Cohen S, Meunier C, et al. Pure red cell aplasia and associated thymoma. Clin Pract 2011;1(1):e1.

31. Chen J, Yang Y, Zhu D, et al. Thymoma with pure red cell aplasia and Good's syndrome. Ann Thorac Surg 2011;91(5):1620–2.

32. Onuki T, Kiyoki Y, Ueda S, et al. Invasive thymoma with pure red cell aplasia and amegakaryocytic thrombocytopenia. Hematol Rep 2016;8(4):6680.

33. Fujishima N, Hirokawa M, Fujishima M, et al. Oligoclonal T cell expansion in blood but not in the thymus from a patient with thymoma-associated pure red cell aplasia. Haematologica 2006;91(12 Suppl):ECR47.

34. Sasidharan PK, Sujith OK, Easaw PC, et al. Pure red cell aplasia associated with thymoma. J Assoc Physicians India 1998;46(3):312–3.

35. Garcia Vela JA, Monteserin MC, Oña F, et al. Cyclosporine A used as a single drug in the treatment of pure red cell aplasia associated with thymoma. Am J Hematol 1993;42(2):238–9.

36. Feinsilber D, Mears KA, Pettiford BL. Polyparaneoplastic manifestations of malignant thymoma: a unique case of myasthenia, autoimmune hepatitis, pure red cell aplasia, and keratoconjunctivitis sicca. Cureus 2017;9(6):e1374.

37. Eridani S, Whitehead S, Sawyer B, et al. Pure red cell aplasia and thymoma: demonstration of persisting inhibition of erythropoiesis after thymectomy and resolution after immune suppressive treatment. Clin Lab Haematol 1986;8(3):181–5.

38. Maeda T, Shiokawa S, Yoshikawa Y, et al. Successful treatment of pure red cell aplasia with cyclosporin A and erythropoietin after thymectomy in a 88-year old woman. Haematologica 2004;89(6 Suppl):ECR17.

39. Larroche C, Mouthon L, Casadevall N, et al. Successful treatment of thymoma-associated pure red cell aplasia with intravenous immunoglobulins. Eur J Haematol 2000;65(1):74–6.

40. Samaiya A, Chumber S, Kashyap R, et al. Pure red cell aplasia with thymoma. J Assoc Physicians India 2001;49:679–80.

41. Sharma K, Kapoor P, Pande JN, et al. Pure red cell aplasia with thymoma. J Assoc Physicians India 1982;30(7):463–5.

42. Krantz SB. Diagnosis and treatment of pure red cell aplasia. Med Clin North Am 1976;60(5):945–58.

43. Anhalt GJ, Kim SC, Stanley JR, et al. Paraneoplastic pemphigus. An autoimmune mucocutaneous disease associated with neoplasia. N Engl J Med 1990;323(25):1729–35.

44. Takeshita K, Amano M, Shimizu T, et al. Thymoma with pemphigus foliaceus. Intern Med 2000;39(9):742–7.

45. Barbetakis N, Samanidis G, Paliouras D, et al. Paraneoplastic pemphigus regression after thymoma resection. World J Surg Oncol 2008;6:83.

46. Winkler DT, Strnad P, Meier ML, et al. Myasthenia gravis, paraneoplastic pemphigus and thymoma, a rare triade. J Neurol 2007;254(11):1601–3.

47. Ascherman DP, Katz P. Systemic lupus erythematosus, pemphigus erythematosus, and thymoma in the same patient. J Clin Rheumatol 1996;2(3):152–5.

48. Yoshida M, Miyoshi T, Sakiyama S, et al. Pemphigus with thymoma improved by thymectomy: report of a case. Surg Today 2013;43(7):806–8.

49. Zheng Y, Cai YZ, Zhang HL, et al. Robotic transsubxiphoid extended thymectomy in a patient with thymoma-associated pemphigus. J Thorac Dis 2017;9(6):E565–9.

50. Reichel A, Benoit S, Giner T, et al. Anti-desmoglein 1 IgG/IgA pemphigus associated with thymoma. J Dtsch Dermatol Ges 2017;15(11):1147–8.

51. Lim JM, Lee SE, Seo J, et al. Paraneoplastic pemphigus associated with a malignant thymoma: a case of persistent and refractory oral ulcerations following thymectomy. Ann Dermatol 2017;29(2):219–22.

52. Fuxiang G, Beutner EH. Pemphigus erythematosus associated with thymoma: a case report. Cutis 1999;64(3):179–82.

53. Lee SE, Hashimoto T, Kim SC. No mucosal involvement in a patient with paraneoplastic pemphigus associated with thymoma and myasthenia gravis. Br J Dermatol 2008;159(4):986–8.

54. Cruz PD Jr, Coldiron BM, Sontheimer RD. Concurrent features of cutaneous lupus erythematosus and pemphigus erythematosus following myasthenia gravis and thymoma. J Am Acad Dermatol 1987;16(2 Pt 2):472–80.

55. Stillman MA, Baer RL. Pemphigus and thymoma. Acta Derm Venereol 1972;52(5):393–7.

56. Rota C, Lupi F, De Pita O, et al. Pemphigus foliaceous with thymoma and multiple comorbidities: a fatal case. Eur J Dermatol 2011;21(3):424–5.

57. Meyer S, Kroiss M, Landthaler M, et al. Thymoma, myasthenia gravis, eruptions of pemphigus vulgaris and a favourable course of relapsing melanoma: an immunological puzzle. Br J Dermatol 2006;155(3):638–40.

58. Evoli A, Lancaster E. Paraneoplastic disorders in thymoma patients. J Thorac Oncol 2014;9(9 Suppl 2):S143–7.

59. Tsivgoulis G, Mikroulis D, Katsanos AH, et al. Paraneoplastic Isaac's syndrome associated with thymoma and anti-neuronal nuclear antibodies 1. J Neurol Sci 2014;343(1–2):245–6.

60. Paul BS, Singh G, Bansal RK, et al. Isaac's syndrome associated with myasthenia gravis and thymoma. Indian J Med Sci 2010;64(7):320–4.

61. Viallard JF, Vincent A, Moreau JF, et al. Thymoma-associated neuromyotonia with antibodies against voltage-gated potassium channels presenting as chronic intestinal pseudo-obstruction. Eur Neurol 2005;53(2):60–3.

62. García-Merino A, Cabello A, Mora JS, et al. Continuous muscle fiber activity, peripheral neuropathy, and thymoma. Ann Neurol 1991;29(2):215–8.

63. Abou-Zeid E, Boursoulian LJ, Metzer WS, et al. Morvan syndrome: a case report and review of the literature. J Clin Neuromuscul Dis 2012;13(4):214–27.

64. Lee EK, Maselli RA, Ellis WG, et al. Morvan's fibrillary chorea: a paraneoplastic manifestation of thymoma. J Neurol Neurosurg Psychiatry 1998;65(6):857–62.

65. Galié E, Renna R, Plantone D, et al. Paraneoplastic Morvan's syndrome following surgical treatment of recurrent thymoma: a case report. Oncol Lett 2016;12(4):2716–9.

66. Agius MA, Zhu S, Lee EK, et al. Antibodies to AChR, synapse-organizing proteins, titin, and other muscle proteins in Morvan's fibrillary chorea. Ann N Y Acad Sci 1998;841:522–4.

67. Maselli RA, Agius M, Lee EK, et al. Morvan's fibrillary chorea. Electrodiagnostic and in vitro microelectrode findings. Ann N Y Acad Sci 1998;841:497–500.

68. Josephs KA, Silber MH, Fealey RD, et al. Neurophysiologic studies in Morvan syndrome. J Clin Neurophysiol 2004;21(6):440–5.

69. Evoli A, Lo Monaco M, Marra R, et al. Multiple paraneoplastic diseases associated with thymoma. Neuromuscul Disord 1999;9(8):601–3.

70. Antozzi C, Frassoni C, Vincent A, et al. Sequential antibodies to potassium channels and glutamic acid decarboxylase in neuromyotonia. Neurology 2005;64(7):1290–3.

71. Kelleher P, Misbah SA. What is Good's syndrome? Immunological abnormalities in patients with thymoma. J Clin Pathol 2003;56(1):12–6.

72. Arend SM, Dik H, van Dissel JT. Good's syndrome: the association of thymoma and hypogammaglobulinemia. Clin Infect Dis 2001;32(2):323–5.

73. Tarr PE, Lucey DR, Infectious Complications of Immunodeficiency with Thymoma (ICIT) Investigators. Good's syndrome: the association of thymoma with immunodeficiency. Clin Infect Dis 2001;33(4):585–6.

74. Soppi E, Eskola J, Röyttä M, et al. Thymoma with immunodeficiency (Good's syndrome) associated with myasthenia gravis and benign IgG gammopathy. Arch Intern Med 1985;145(9):1704–7.

75. Nagoya A, Kanzaki R, Nakagiri T, et al. Ectopic cervical thymoma accompanied by Good's syndrome. Ann Thorac Cardiovasc Surg 2014;20(Suppl):531–4.

76. DeBoard ZM, Taylor BJ. Good's syndrome: successful management of thymoma with hypoimmunoglobulinemia. Ann Thorac Surg 2015;100(5):1903–5.

77. Hon C, Chui WH, Cheng LC, et al. Thymoma associated with keratoconjunctivitis, lichen planus, hypogammaglobinemia, and absent circulating B cells. J Clin Oncol 2006;24(18):2960–1.

78. Verne GN, Amann ST, Cosgrove C, et al. Chronic diarrhea associated with thymoma and hypogammaglobulinemia (Good's syndrome). South Med J 1997;90(4):444–6.

79. Oshikiri T, Morikawa T, Sugiura H, et al. Thymoma associated with hypogammaglobulinemia (Good's syndrome): report of a case. Surg Today 2002;32(3):264–6.

80. de Jesus NP, Carvalho PM, Dias FM, et al. Dementia in a patient with thymoma and hypogammaglobulinaemia (Good's syndrome). Cases J 2008;1(1):90.

81. Khan S, Campbell A, Hunt C, et al. Lichen planus in a case of Good's syndrome (thymoma and immunodeficiency). Interact Cardiovasc Thorac Surg 2009;9(2):345–6.

82. Liu SC, Wang CH. Multiple head and neck tuberculosis granulomas in a patient with thymoma and immunodeficiency (Good's syndrome). Otolaryngol Head Neck Surg 2010;142(3):454–5.

83. Kikuchi R, Mino N, Okamoto T, et al. A case of Good's syndrome: a rare acquired immunodeficiency associated with thymoma. Ann Thorac Cardiovasc Surg 2011;17(1):74–6.

84. Habib AM, Thornton H, Sewell WC, et al. Good's syndrome: is thymectomy the solution? Case report and literature review. Asian Cardiovasc Thorac Ann 2016;24(7):712–4.

85. Ternavasio-de la Vega HG, Velasco-Tirado V, Pozo-Rosado L, et al. Persistence of immunological alterations after thymectomy in Good's syndrome: a clue to its pathogenesis. Cytometry B Clin Cytom 2011;80(5):339–42.

86. Bobbio A, Vescovi P, Ampollini L, et al. Oral erosive lichen planus regression after thymoma resection. Ann Thorac Surg 2007;83(3):1197–9.

87. Mineo TC, Biancari F, D'Andrea V. Myasthenia gravis, psychiatric disturbances, idiopathic thrombocytopenic purpura, and lichen planus associated with cervical thymoma. J Thorac Cardiovasc Surg 1996;111(2):486–7.

88. Aronson IK, Soltani K, Paik KI, et al. Triad of lichen planus, myasthenia gravis, and thymoma. Arch Dermatol 1978;114(2):255–8.

89. Motegi S, Uchiyama A, Yamada K, et al. Lichen planus complicated with thymoma: report of three Japanese cases and review of the published work. J Dermatol 2015;42(11):1072–7.

90. Hayashi A, Shiono H, Okumura M. Thymoma accompanied by lichen planus. Interact Cardiovasc Thorac Surg 2008;7(2):347–8.

91. Calista D. Oral erosive lichen planus associated with thymoma. Int J Dermatol 2001;40(12):762–4.

92. Ng PP, Ng SK, Chng HH. Pemphigus foliaceus and oral lichen planus in a patient with systemic lupus erythematosus and thymoma. Clin Exp Dermatol 1998;23(4):181–4.

93. Lee BW, Ihm SH, Shin HS, et al. Malignant thymoma associated with myasthenia gravis, Graves' disease, and SIADH. Intern Med 2008;47(11):1009–12.

94. Matsumoto Y, Hirai S, Ohashi M, et al. Sjögren's syndrome associated with thymoma. J Am Acad Dermatol 1996;35(4):639–40.

95. Fujiu K, Kanno R, Shio Y, et al. Triad of thymoma, myasthenia gravis and pure red cell aplasia combined with Sjögren's syndrome. Jpn J Thorac Cardiovasc Surg 2004;52(7):345–8.

96. Tsai Y, Lin Y, Chen C, et al. Thymoma associated with myasthenia gravis and Sjögren syndrome. West Indian Med J 2013;62(3):264–5.

97. Ben-Shahar M, Rosenblatt E, Green J, et al. Malignant thymoma associated with progressive systemic sclerosis. Am J Med Sci 1987;294(4):262–7.

98. Padda SK, Yao X, Antonicelli A, et al. Paraneoplastic syndromes and thymic malignancies: an examination of the International Thymic Malignancy Interest Group retrospective database. J Thorac Oncol 2018;13(3):436–46.

99. Milne JA, Anderson JR, MacSween RN, et al. Thymectomy in acute systemic lupus erythematosus and rheumatoid arthritis. Br Med J 1967;1(5538):461–4.

100. Szobor A, Molnár J. Effect of thymectomy in immune diseases other than myasthenia. Acta Med Hung 1985;42(3–4):101–8.

101. Szobor A. Benefit of thymectomy in immune diseases other than myasthenia. Lancet 1984;1(8371):277–8.

102. Tellez-Zenteno JF, Remes-Troche JM, Mimenza-Alvarado A, et al. The association of myasthenia gravis and connective tissue diseases. Effects of thymectomy in six cases with rheumatoid arthritis and one case with systemic lupus erythematosus. Neurologia 2003;18(2):54–8.

103. Weiner HL. Multiple sclerosis is an inflammatory T-cell-mediated autoimmune disease. Arch Neurol 2004;61(10):1613–5.

104. D'Andrea V, Meco G, Corvese F, et al. The role of the thymus in multiple sclerosis. Ital J Neurol Sci 1989;10(1):43–8.

105. Roach ES. Is multiple sclerosis an autoimmune disorder? Arch Neurol 2004;61(10):1615–6.

106. Ferguson TB, Clifford DB, Montgomery EB, et al. Thymectomy in multiple sclerosis. Two preliminary trials. J Thorac Cardiovasc Surg 1983;85(1):88–93.

107. Trotter JL, Clifford DB, Montgomery EB, et al. Thymectomy in multiple sclerosis: a 3-year follow-up. Neurology 1985;35(7):1049–51.

108. Veĭn AM, Khomak VI, Belokrinitskiĭ DV, et al. Thymectomy in disseminated sclerosis. Sov Med 1981;12:42–5.

109. Finnie IA, Shields R, Sutton R, et al. Crohn's disease and myasthenia gravis: a possible role for thymectomy. Gut 1994;35(2):278–9.

110. Lane RJM, Hudgson R. Thymectomy in polymyositis. Lancet 1984;1(8377):626–7.

111. Evoli A, Minicuci GM, Vitaliani R, et al. Paraneoplastic diseases associated with thymoma. J Neurol 2007;254(6):756–62.

112. Raschilas F, Mouthon L, André MH, et al. Concomitant polymyositis and myasthenia gravis reveal malignant thymoma. A case report and review of the literature. Ann Med Interne (Paris) 1999;150(5):370–3.

113. Lee AB, Thurston RS. Malignant thymoma and myasthenia gravis presenting as polymyositis: a case report. J La State Med Soc 2008;160(5):286–8.

114. Souadjian JV, Howell LP, Lambert EH. Thymoma with myopathy. Report of a case. Minn Med 1969;52(4):595–6.

115. Klein JJ, Gottlieb AJ, Mones RJ, et al. Thymoma and polymyositis. Onset of myasthenia gravis after thymectomy: report of two cases. Arch Intern Med 1964;113:142–52.

116. Lin J, Lu J, Zhao C, et al. Giant cell polymyositis associated with myasthenia gravis and thymoma. J Clin Neurosci 2014;21(12):2252–4.

117. Cumming WJ. Thymectomy in refractory dermatomyositis. Muscle Nerve 1989;12(5):424.

118. Ago T, Nakamura M, Iwata I, et al. Dermatomyositis associated with invasive thymoma. Intern Med 1999;38(2):155–9.

119. Suzuki K, Inomata M, Shiraishi S, et al. Thymoma with autoimmune hemolytic anemia. Case Rep Oncol 2014;7(3):764–8.

120. Tuncer Elmaci N, Ratip S, Ince-Günal D, et al. Myasthenia gravis with thymoma and autoimmune haemolytic anaemia. A case report. Neurol Sci 2003;24(1):34–6.

121. Halperin IC, Minogue WF, Komninos ZD. Autoimmune hemolytic anemia and myasthenia gravis associated with thymoma. N Engl J Med 1966; 275(12):663–4.

122. Rennenberg RJ, Pauwels P, Vlasveld LT. A case of thymoma-associated autoimmune haemolytic anaemia. Neth J Med 1997;50(3):110–4.

123. De Keyzer K, Peeters P, Verhelst C, et al. Autoimmune haemolytic anaemia associated with a thymoma: case report and review of the literature. Acta Clin Belg 2009;64(5):447–51.

124. Arntzenius AB, Bieger R. Disappearance of autoantibody-induced haemolysis after excision of a malignant thymoma. Neth J Med 1991;38(3–4): 117–21.

125. Rubinstein I, Langevitz P, Hirsch R, et al. Autoimmune hemolytic anemia as the presenting manifestation of malignant thymoma. Acta Haematol 1985; 74(1):40–2.

126. Kornfeld P, Glass J, Papatestas AE, et al. Case report: thymectomy-induced remission of acquired autoimmune hemolytic anemia in an adult with myasthenia gravis. Am J Med Sci 1979;277(1): 111–6.

127. Hirooka M, Yoshioka K, Ono T, et al. Autoimmune hemolytic anemia in a child treated with thymectomy. Tohoku J Exp Med 1970;101(3):227–35.

128. Wilmers MJ, Russell PA. Autoimmune haemolytic anaemia in an infant treated by thymectomy. Lancet 1963;2(7314):915–7.

129. Karaklis A, Valaes T, Pantelakis SN, et al. Thymectomy in an infant with autoimmune haemolytic anaemia. Lancet 1964;2(7363):778–80.

130. Webb HW, Wilkinson AH Jr, David JK. Autoimmune hemolytic anemia: successful treatment by thymectomy. J Pediatr Surg 1974;9(5):771–4.

131. Johnson CA, Abildgaard CF. Treatment of idiopathic autoimmune hemolytic anemia in children.

Review and report of two fatal cases in infancy. Acta Paediatr Scand 1976;65(3):375–9.

132. Oski FA, Abelson NM. Autoimmune hemolytic anemia in an infant. Report of a case treated unsuccessfully with thymectomy. J Pediatr 1965;67(5): 752–8.

133. Shelly S, Agmon-Levin N, Altman A, et al. Thymoma and autoimmunity. Cell Mol Immunol 2011; 8(3):199–202.

134. Boonen A, Rennenberg R, van der Linden S. Thymoma-associated systemic lupus erythematosus, exacerbating after thymectomy. A case report and review of the literature. Rheumatology (Oxford) 2000;39(9):1044–6.

135. Jang SJ, Wu YC, Chuang WY, et al. Impending cardiac tamponade as the initial presentation of thymoma in a systemic lupus erythematosus patient. Lupus 2010;19(3):337–40.

136. Larsson O. Thymoma and systemic lupus erythematosus in the same patient. Lancet 1963; 2(7309):665–6.

137. Menon S, Snaith ML, Isenberg DA. The association of malignancy with SLE: an analysis of 150 patients under long-term review. Lupus 1993;2(3):177–81.

138. Zandman-Goddard G, Lorber M, Shoenfeld Y. Systemic lupus erythematosus and thymoma–a double-edged sword. Int Arch Allergy Immunol 1995;108(1):99–102.

139. Simeone JF, McCloud T, Putman CE, et al. Thymoma and systemic lupus erythematosus. Thorax 1975;30(6):697–700.

140. Bozzolo E, Bellone M, Quaroni N, et al. Thymoma associated with systemic lupus erythematosus and immunologic abnormalities. Lupus 2000;9(2):151–4.

141. Mastaglia FL, Papadimitriou JM, Dawkins RL, et al. Vacuolar myopathy associated with chloroquine, lupus erythematosus and thymoma. Report of a case with unusual mitochondrial changes and lipid accumulation in muscle. J Neurol Sci 1977;34(3): 315–28.

142. Duchmann R, Schwarting A, Poralla T, et al. Thymoma and pure red cell aplasia in a patient with systemic lupus erythematosus. Scand J Rheumatol 1995;24(4):251–4.

143. Claudy AL, Touraine JL, Schmitt D, et al. Thymoma and lupus erythematosus. Report of 3 cases. Thymus 1983;5(3–4):209–22.

144. Steven MM, Westedt ML, Eulderink F, et al. Systemic lupus erythematosus and invasive thymoma: report of two cases. Ann Rheum Dis 1984;43(6): 825–8.

145. Mackay IR, Smalley M. Results of thymectomy in systemic lupus erythematosus: observations on clinical course and serological reactions. Clin Exp Immunol 1966;1(2):129–38.

146. Tsuchiya M. Immunological abnormalities involving the thymus in ulcerative colitis and therapeutic

effects of thymectomy. Gastroenterol Jpn 1984; 19(3):232–46.

147. Tsuchiya M, Hibi T, Watanabe M, et al. Thymectomy in ulcerative colitis: a report of cases over a 13 year period. Thymus 1991;17(2):67–73.

148. Okubo K, Kondo N, Okamoto T, et al. Excision of an invasive thymoma: a cure for ulcerative colitis? Ann Thorac Surg 2001;71(6):2013–5.

149. Deeb ME, Brinster CJ, Kucharzuk J, et al. Expanded indications for transcervical thymectomy in the management of anterior mediastinal masses. Ann Thorac Surg 2001;72(1):208–11.

150. Burt BM, Yao X, Shrager J, et al. Determinants of complete resection of thymoma by minimally invasive and open thymectomy: analysis of an international registry. J Thorac Oncol 2017;12(1):129–36.

Moving?

Make sure your subscription moves with you!

To notify us of your new address, find your **Clinics Account Number** (located on your mailing label above your name), and contact customer service at:

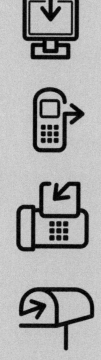

Email: journalscustomerservice-usa@elsevier.com

800-654-2452 (subscribers in the U.S. & Canada)
314-447-8871 (subscribers outside of the U.S. & Canada)

Fax number: 314-447-8029

Elsevier Health Sciences Division
Subscription Customer Service
3251 Riverport Lane
Maryland Heights, MO 63043

Printed and bound by CPI Group (UK) Ltd, Croydon, CR0 4YY

08/05/2025

01864745-0015